Dedication

 This book is dedicated to sweet baby James. You have forever changed the person that I am. You have forever changed the lives of so many who love you. Your joy is immeasurable. Your love reaches places that most of us cannot go.

Preface

First of all, thank you for taking the time to read this book. I wrote this as a small glimpse inside the heart of a mom, raising a boy with high needs, and the ups and downs along the way. I wanted to write honestly; about my journey, the pain, grief, the joy, and learning to embrace the stages.
What I have written is going to be uncomfortably honest. It is the thoughts that most of us keep hidden forever. The things we would never dare give voice to. I am predicting that I am going to feel very uncomfortable when someone tells me that they have read my book. They will now know me in a way that I maybe wouldn't have chosen; it is almost like you are standing naked in front of someone, waiting for the criticism (and you don't want to see me naked!). So why write it then? And more so, why publish it? The answer is so simple. Too many people are walking so alone. Too many people feel trapped and don't know how to reach out. Let me reach out to you.
I started to write this book as a way to share my heart's journey with other girls, women, and moms. We all walk different paths, but our hearts go through the same processes. And even more specifically, to connect with

those who have walked the path of raising a child who has faced challenges far beyond what we ever thought would come into our lives. As we learn to share with honesty and be genuine with one another, the curtains fall, the walls crumble down around us, the loneliness that so often invades our hearts starts to warm up slightly. Our journeys become easier when we realize that we are not alone. Once we start to truly see that our hearts are feeling the same emotions and hurts and joys, we can learn from each other's valleys and triumphs. And maybe once we start to see each other for our hearts, the judgement will slowly drop away.

Women don't meet the way that they used to. They used to carve time into their regular schedules to meet intentionally; sharing life's triumphs and burdens with one another. Somewhere, amidst our hectic lives, we have lost this valuable tradition. So many of our encounters are made up of surface level small talk as we rush on to the next scheduled activity. We don't allow our lives the space to create those deep friendships that open our hearts and give the freedom for complete honesty in the midst of our trials. We miss the aches of others hearts. Our hearts remain suppressed, and we are missing out on that safety to speak our hearts and find understanding and acceptance despite the ugliness of our reality.

My hope is that this book is a place for us to meet. To set aside everything hectic, to set aside the need to uphold the perfect standard that is expected as we rush by someone, answering that we are good, of course. I've expressed my heart very honestly, in the midst of the biggest trial life may ever hand me, in the hopes that someone else will feel less alone, whether our paths are similar, or our hearts are both aching while walking different roads.

I am 6 years into my journey, and I still struggle. I will always struggle. It will never go away. It will only change. My struggle has become easier, only because my heart has changed. My heart has become softer, and more calloused. I've become more sensitive, and less susceptible, yet more compassionate. My heart has learned the value in taking risks, and the significance of stepping back. I've allowed myself the space to process, to accept, and to challenge. My struggle has also become harder. The challenges are not dissolving with my new strength and courage and compassion, they are increasing. I am learning that they will always be increasing.

    People often say that once you become a parent you forever wear your heart on the outside. You feel things with an intensity and fierceness that you never could have imagined before. Now imagine if the intensity and fierceness was for a child that was forever vulnerable, who was at the mercy of their circumstances and the people surrounding them in every moment. A child who was unable to communicate with you when they felt hurt, sad, angry, left out, or different.

    I spend my days, every single day, weighing the decisions I have made; did James really get enough to eat? Did he go to school hungry? Does he get cared for properly on the bus? It's quite cold today.... is he staying warm enough? Is anyone checking his diaper? Is that substitute aide at school being kind and loving with him? Is she laughing with him? Does he feel hurt today but can't tell me? He was crying so much and I put him to bed early... maybe he was trying to tell me that something hurts? Or that he's feeling angry? Maybe sad? Is he starting to notice how different he is from everyone else? Is he starting to show signs of anxiety or depression over not being able to get his body to do what he so desperately wants it to do, and I am somehow missing all the signs? It doesn't end. This happens every day. All day.

    I began writing this book when James was six years old, and I finished when he was eight years old. You will notice different parts of the story are written at different stages. You will see changes in my heart, my strengths, my daily struggles. But you will see far more similarities. Our childhood stages last much longer and cycle much slower than most families.

  I have shared our story, sometimes in chronological order, but with a lot of the gaps filled in later on in stories about my heart. You will get a very real look at the day to day life caring for a disabled child, along with how the heart journeys through this. You will find some email updates I sent out to friends and family in our early stages in the book, as well as a few blog entries I wrote when James was three years old. I have included these because they are the only writings that I have from when I was in the middle of it all.

  Sometimes people ask me what it is like raising James, and I never really have an answer. How do I sum that up in a two minute conversation? If I only have a few minutes, my answer is going be joy. This child has brought me joy far deeper than I ever could have imagined. What I don't say is how much it hurts. It hurts to love a child who you know you will likely bury one day. It hurts to love a child who is faced with limitations every single day. Limitations that he understands, and fights, but cannot win. It hurts to love a child that you don't fully know the way the a parent should know their child.

  Caring for James has become so much of who I am, that I fear the day where I do not have him. Who will I be? What will be left of me? Will I know how to carry on when I am no longer defined by being a caregiver? Will my personality change too much? Will I keep my compassion, or will that fade with the pain? He changed me so much when he came into my life, and I fear how I may change if I have to let him go.

As Long As It's Healthy...

October 22, 2007, I gave birth to a little boy. A beautiful little boy that completed our perfect little family of mom, dad, daughter, and now son. A little boy that would terrorize his little sister, play baseball with his dad, play outside all day with his friends, coming inside covered in mud, and tracking it throughout the house. A handsome teenage boy who would walk across his graduation stage, and have our full support to follow his dreams, whatever they may be. A young man that would bring home girls to meet his mom, until one day we welcomed one of those beautiful girls into our family forever. However, that little boy was whisked off to NICU after spending only minutes in my arms.

After 11 days in the neonatal intensive care unit we would discover that James was born with something called cCMV, congenital cytomegalovirus. This is a virus that I would have contracted early on in my pregnancy, without knowing, and passed on to my baby.

We have all grown up in a world where the words "as long as it's healthy" have become cliché. "We don't care if it's a girl or a boy, just as long as it's healthy." Most of us with children have uttered these words at some point in our lives. Most grandparents have spoken these words in anticipation of the new grandbaby. And likely, they have shattered somebody's heart without any intent of doing so. Is the most important thing really that we have a healthy baby? Isn't that the ideal? Absolutely. Absolutely, without any doubt or hesitation, all babies should have a healthy start in life. Never in our wildest imagination would we want a child to suffer. But let me tell you, the most important thing is not that that child is healthy. It's that that child is accepted, loved, and nurtured.

    James is six years old right now. And I've found my heart consistently breaking over the last few months. I've known since the first year of his life that I would one day write about my hearts journey through this, but I have barely written a page of it down, until now. Journaling was recommended to me time and time again, by so many people, as a way of coping. As a way to let out my true, ugly, scary feelings, in a way that wouldn't push anyone away from me, but would still be therapeutic. I am not writing this book from old journal entries, because I don't have any. I could never bear to write out my honest feelings, because they were so raw and real, that I couldn't stand to see it. My true thoughts were terrifying at many times; far too shocking to possibly share with another person, or even write on paper.

    My feelings are still raw from time to time, but my heart has healed. Our circumstances have not changed, but my heart can now find a way through it all, even though some days it is still broken. I've learned to allow myself to not be okay when I need to not be okay. That doesn't mean I fall apart and withdraw from the world for that time. It means that in my heart, I can now allow myself to break, while still being compassionate and loving. Those closest to me can feel the subtle differences when I'm allowing myself to feel the struggle, but most people would never know. Not because I am trying to put on an act, but because this is my journey. And if you step into my world and my heart I will let you in and be quite honest, but most people do not have a clue what the heart of a parent with a high needs child goes through, and therefore, unsolicited sharing of my heart breaking often leads to sympathy, which is not at all what I am needing. And some of you are nodding your heads and possibly letting a tear fall right now, as this is your heart and your life. And others are saying, "but if you don't tell us we won't know". And yes, while this is true, I've learned discernment when it comes to sharing. I'm a very open and genuine person, and if I feel that I'm being met there, I am an open book.

My heart has been breaking lately for the stage that James is in. He is six years old, and in grade one. When my daughter, Julia, was six, she was always off to a birthday party, or running in and out of the house with friends. James is six, and in the last 3 years, he has been invited to one birthday party. ONE. And we went. The little girl that invited him came and said hi to him, but then carried on with her friends who could run. One child there spent a lot of her time with him. We put him on a scooter and she pulled him around the gymnasium, while he squealed with delight, often so high pitched that you couldn't even hear him. She would just sit beside him and hold his hand when he was in his wheelchair. But obviously, since she was 5, she also left several times to run. And James cried.

All the parents stayed at this party, and not one of them acknowledged James, or myself. At one point I prayed so hard that my tears would not fall, but my eyes were so full. I was already sitting all alone, I did not also want to have tears falling off my face.

And this is what is so very hard to explain to people. This is not a jealousy issue. In no way has this ever been a jealousy issue, nor will it ever be a jealousy issue. I am not jealous of your child who can walk and talk and eat. I am not jealous that as a parent you got a healthy baby and I did not. This is not what is going through my mind as I sit at this birthday party and fight back the tears with every ounce of strength that I can find. What is breaking my heart, is watching my son want so badly to be a part of everything just like everyone else. What breaks my heart is watching James' eyes, as he watches those parents interact with all the children who are running and laughing, and purposefully avoid him.

James loves so unconditionally. He is fascinated by everything and everyone around him. He is also fully aware of what is going on at all times. He knows when you walk around him, and avoid eye contact. He knows when you talk to every other child but refuse to look into his eyes, because you know he cannot say words back to you. So instead you avoid any discomfort you may feel and simply do not acknowledge him. He knows when you hand every child a treat but you simply walk by him, because he can't eat that sucker. So instead you choose not to acknowledge that there is a little boy who cannot take his eyes off you, expectantly waiting, because you did just give every child there a sucker, so why would he assume that he is any different. And then he realizes that it's like he doesn't exist. He makes a loud noise, and bites his hands, but everyone looks away, because it might be awkward if you saw the hurt and confusion in his eyes, because you have no intention of coming anywhere near him. This is why my eyes fill with tears, and often those tears barely even touch my face before they hit the floor.

So that was the ONE birthday party that James has been invited to in the last three years. And while it was heartbreaking, I would still say yes in a heartbeat to any and every other invitation. Why? Because while most of us remember the hurt of an experience and try to avoid further hurt or embarrassment, James does not. He simply loves. He loves people and children and pets and music and sunshine and fresh air and loud music and fun and water and treats, and most of all, love. He loves when someone takes the time to make eye contact with him, to touch his hand or his face, to have a little conversation with him. He loves being included in what everyone else is doing., even if he is simply sitting in his wheelchair observing and laughing along with everyone else. And I will do everything I can to provide him with these opportunities and allow him to be with people.

James is eight years old now, and hasn't been invited to another party since.

It's a boy!

James' birth was three weeks early, and objectionably fast! We went back to Saskatoon to spend Thanksgiving weekend with family, and were on our way home, to Caronport, Saskatchewan, on October 22. We were just leaving my parents house, van all loaded up with my husband and I, Julia who was two years old, and our rottweiler Grace. We stopped to see my mother in law at the hotel where she works on our way out of the city. Getting out of the van I was starting to feel a little funny, and by the time we were in the lobby I remember leaning on the front desk, and my mother in law said to get me to the hospital now – I was in labor! We figured I had some time since Julia's birth was much slower; however, the pain was intensifying rather quickly. I called a friend to see if I could drop my daughter off there before we went to the hospital, but by the time I had her on the phone I had to hand it to my husband to talk to her, because I couldn't talk through the pain any longer! She said of course, so we drove about ten minutes back to my parents to drop off Grace, who likely wouldn't be welcomed at the hospital with us! By the time we got there I was yelling at John to get her out and get me to the hospital – this baby was coming! You just know when you are playing with fate, and you are running out of time. From there we had to go straight to the hospital, there was no time to drop Julia off.

    The drive to the hospital took about ten minutes, in morning rush hour traffic, with me wretchedly screaming at John to run every red light we encountered. I was lifting myself off the van seat, and squeezing with every ounce of strength I could find, as I could feel the baby's head crowning and touching the seat! I was screaming like someone was killing me, John was driving like someone who had no idea how critical it was that he speed up and run the stupid red lights already, and poor sweet Julia was in her car seat in the middle row of our minivan, asking if mommy was going to be okay! Thank goodness she has no memories from this day.

    We got to the hospital, parked outside the emergency room doors at Royal University Hospital, and the second I stood up my water broke. So off I went, hobbling through those hospital doors, yelling that I was having a baby, soaked from the waist down. Let me tell you, they get you a stretcher awfully fast when you make that kind of an entrance!

    John was taking Julia out of the van while the doctors put me on a stretcher, threw a sheet over me, and were running me towards the elevator, stating that I WOULD NOT be having this baby in emergency, using that super annoying condescending authoritative voice that a young child would be scolded with, as if that would make me go "oh ok, silly me, I'll just hold this baby in until you say it is okay to have it." Not quite. I was screaming back that the baby was already half out! The doctor very matter of factly told me that the baby was not half out. Which was when, in my most tactful moment, I lifted the sheet and screamed that YES in fact, the baby was half out. Well, looks like I was correct, because he started running back towards the emergency department with me, but I had James with no assistance before we even reached a room.

And finally, in walks John. James was already over on another table, surrounded by so many doctors, and I had several doctors and nurses around me as well. Julia stayed with the nurse at the front desk, and John called someone to come and get her. My whole body was convulsing from the trauma of delivering so fast; they covered me with multiple hot blankets and gave me meds immediately to try to stop it. It took a few doses of meds, but soon my body stopped convulsing and I could lie still and pay more attention to what was all going on around me. I'm not sure what I all said, or rather shouted, in the heat of the delivery, but I do know that John came in and apologized on my behalf. Haha.

After some time, they put me in a wheelchair, and they gently laid my baby in my arms for the very first time, and we already knew that his name was James.

Little James Elzar Patterson. 6lbs of perfect.

Once up on maternity, I tried to breast feed, which he was not interested in yet, so they sent me for a shower. My body was still fairly shaky, so the nurse helped me onto the stool in the shower, and I slowly got cleaned up. I got myself out, and slowly walked out clinging to my iv pole for stability, just in time to see them transferring James' tiny body into an enclosed isolet. I asked what was happening, and they said they were taking James up to the NICU for observation. I started to fall, faint, but my nurse caught me and got me back into bed.

And just like that, it was just me, in ugly hospital clothes, still shaking, and no baby to hold. I wasn't scared at this point though. I wasn't really told anything, other than he needed a little bit of observation. I figured I would still be bringing him home when I was discharged, so I was going to get myself looking human again and get some sleep! John went and got some food, and brought me some clean clothes, because I wasn't going to lie around in hospital clothes with no baby to hold. Delivering that fast is incredibly hard on your body, but once the convulsing was gone, I was almost back to normal. The after contractions felt much worse than when I delivered much slower with Julia, but with no epidural this time, there was no tearing and no recovery time. Since I was feeling so good, it was incredibly boring to be stuck in the hospital with no baby. Because we were from out of town, they kept me there as long as they could so I would be closer to where James was.

The two days that I spent on the maternity ward got hard. They ended up feeling like an eternity. The NICU only let me come down to see James a few times a day, and no one could tell me when he was being discharged or what was going on. The NICU doctors had nothing to tell the nurses on the maternity ward, so I just kept getting the run around.

October 30, 2007, as I was standing at James' isolet in the NICU in Royal University Hospital, during Dr's rounds, I finally found out what was wrong with my baby. For the last 8 days they had been running test after test on his tiny little body, and then on me, completely puzzled by what was causing his symptoms. His platelets were very low. He had a bumpy red rash all over his body. He was jaundiced. He could not control his body temperature. His tiny frail body tremored for no apparent reason. He was born weighing 6lbs, and had now gone down below 5lbs. His head was so small it didn't even register on the charts. He hardly slept. His stools were ghostly white and a weird consistency. His birth had been so fast that I actually delivered him with no assistance in the emergency room hallway on a stretcher.

This morning, one neonatologist, about six interns, and the head of nursing in the NICU unit circled around

James' tiny isolet. The nurse took my hand and quietly said that they had some answers, and after the doctor left she would sit with me and explain it much better. The doctor said a bunch of big words that went entirely over my head, all I remember of what he said was the ending. He said, "your son will most likely become deaf and blind in the first eight years of his life, but other than that he will be just fine. We will keep him here for about two more nights and then you are free to go home with your baby."

My baby was going to go deaf and blind? Both? Why? The nurse must have led me to a chair and sat me down because I do not remember going with her. My world had narrowed into a dark corridor. I took a few breaths, and looked up to see a very compassionate lady looking back at me. From there she explained to me that James was born with congenital cytamegolovirus, known as cCMV. She wrote it on a small slip of pink paper for me to take with when we were done, because I obviously was not taking in all that she was saying. We talked about my pregnancy, had I been sick? I was so confused because my pregnancy was perfect. I loved every minute of being pregnant this time. I had a cold at the beginning of my pregnancy, but only a mild cold. Nothing I took any medicine for or stayed home from work for, just a normal cold virus. That was it. That cold, which was actually CMV, transmitted to my baby within the first few weeks of pregnancy. And now he was going to go deaf and blind. The nurse walked me to the family waiting room where there were some books I could read more about this in. I sank into the black reclining chair, with two enormous medical books, and sat by myself reading, until it was time to go pump again.

Neo natal Intensive Care Unit

I was discharged two nights after having had James, but because he was still in the NICU, and we lived over 2 hours away from Saskatoon, they allowed me to sleep in what is called a parents room just down the hallway from the NICU. It was just a normal hospital room with four beds and a bathroom, and most of the time I had the room to myself. I spent most of my time in the NICU, except during the times that even parents weren't allowed in the unit. Then I would spend some time in the waiting room in the nice comfortable leather chairs and couches. Well as comfortable as hospital couches can be, but they sure beat my tiny hard bed that I spent the remainder of my time on. If I wasn't in the unit sitting beside James, I could often be found in the pumping room. A little room, with two rocking chairs and curtains in between, and the horridly loud hospital breast pumps, where other moms like me, who were sleep deprived, worried, lonely, scared, and hungry, were trying to pump enough milk so that when our babies were strong enough they could try breastfeeding! For now, we were pumping hard, and handing it off to the nurses for bottle feeding. I usually only had an ounce or two; how embarrassing to walk in to hand them only a few drops really in the bottom of the huge container they kept giving me to fill. Could they not have given me a smaller container so I at least felt like just maybe I was accomplishing something? I had just sat in a gross little room for an hour, being milked by pitifully loud pumps. Anyone walking by in the hallway could hear them going. And I did this for an hour, every three hours, only to hand them a few ounces.

NICU was a place that terrified me while we were there. They had my baby, and I had to call into the unit from a little black phone in the waiting room, to ask permission to see my baby. Then I had to stand at huge stainless steel sinks and scrub my hands, fingers and arms for two minutes before I could enter. The first day that James occupied his little isolet, we could hold him for brief periods still. I even got to try breastfeeding. His suck was really too weak to get anything, but I tried. By day two he wasn't able to control his temperature well enough any longer and he was hooked up to too many monitors to be able to hold him anymore. I could simply come in, sit down beside him, and occasionally open the little circular hole in the side and sneak a touch while no one was around. Once in a while a nurse would let me put both hands in and change his diaper, which was enormous on him, or even prop his tiny head up with one hand and bottle feed him with the other.

The nurses did not want me in the NICU for feeding times. He could not suck hard enough to get any milk from breastfeeding, so I was pumping, which as I told you was almost a joke, and supplementing with formula, all from a bottle. The tiniest cutest little NICU bottles. They looked like the bottles I had for my doll when I was a little girl. The nurses were so busy that they would often feed him late, and he was dropping too much weight, but they still did not want me in there to do the feeding. I was in the way. I complied for the first few days, but seriously, after your baby has been taken away, you don't yet know what's wrong, they are kicking you out constantly to run test after test after test with no answers, you are living on the occasional snack you run down to the cafeteria to grab and almost no sleep, you haven't showered in days, your husband and daughter are not with you at the hospital, and you are absolutely terrified, a switch seems to flip once you are finally pushed too far.

One evening I very politely told the evening nurse that I was going to sleep for about an hour, but to please wake me to do the next feeding; I felt it was very important for our bonding that I start to do the feedings, and I was more than capable of doing so; I no longer wanted them feeding him. She agreed and I went for a nap. Instead of waking me to feed him, they fed him early, so that they wouldn't have to have me in there, in their way. I woke up after an hour, call it mother's intuition, and went back to his isolet, only to be informed that they had just finished feeding him. Switch officially flipped. Who the hell were they to disobey my instructions? Yes nurses, I so get that you are busy. And I so get that you know what you are doing. But that was MY baby. It's your job, but my baby. I freaked. Right there in the NICU. Yelling, tears, cursing, passion, anger, sadness, confusion. I couldn't even begin to try to tell you what was all said, because I had so much adrenaline pumping through my body in those moments that I literally have zero memory of it. However, I heard it was pretty memorable!

The nursing supervisor on that night came in moments later and apologized profusely, and switched my nurse for the remainder of the night. Very clear signs were made for his isolet that his mother was always to be doing the feedings. The head of nursing arranged a meeting with me for the next day to discuss what had all happened. An official complaint was filed, I was sincerely apologized to, treated with genuine compassion, and respect was given to my wishes. That was the first light bulb moment that I can remember having.

The first moment where I realized I had what it took to raise this child.

To love him through whatever it was that lied ahead for us. To fight for him. And that's such a fine line; where do you burn the bridge and get it done, where do you bite your tongue and cool off first, what do you push for and what do you let slide? Your heart teaches you along the way, you just learn to trust yourself. As long as you keep your heart soft, which is sometimes the hardest part, the rest follows naturally. Not easily, but naturally.

My days with James in the NICU felt lonesome and very long. I went from sitting beside his isolet, to feeding and changing him through those two tiny round holes in the sides of the isolet, to pumping my embarrassing amount of milk to put in the NICU fridge, to taking a quick washroom and stretch break, maybe send off a few texts, and back to sitting beside that isolet. Blood tests were being ran constantly, ultrasounds of his entire body were done, monitors were hooked up, all looking for the cause of the problem. Slowly things started to improve. He began regulating his own temperature, and the top of the isolet was taken off. I was able to hold my baby again! That is a feeling I could never describe. After days of worry and stress and tears, while we still knew nothing, I could feel him against me again. Soon he was strong enough to try breastfeeding again. He was absolutely horrific at it, but we tried, and supplemented with a bottle. His bowel movements became normal, and he started to put on weight again. His rash started to clear up. And then the news of cCMV came.

The morning after the diagnosis an audiologist came up to the NICU and performed a hearing test on James, and his hearing was perfect. A few simple eye tests were done and everything looked good. They gave me slips for follow up audiology and optometrist appointments, an appointment to see the neonatologist in six months, and were discharged from the NICU on November 2, 2007. We put our tiny little 5lb baby boy in the car seat, and got to leave as a family!

I have often been asked since leaving this part of our journey behind, how to best support a family who has a child in NICU, or PICU, or really just in the hospital in general. Here are a few really practical ways that you could offer your support.

- o If you are close with the family, arrange a time to stop at the hospital with a hug, a card with an encouraging note, some healthy snacks, and something to read. They likely won't touch the reading material, but it is there if they could use the distraction. Do not stay longer than a few minutes. They will likely be too polite to ask you to leave, or to admit how tired they are, but simply offer what you brought and be on your way. Texting ahead of time to arrange a time is also vital. Very few times did I leave the ward, and I always wanted to be there for feedings, changing, bathing and doctor rounds.
- o Arrange to simply drop off a card for them, containing some money for meals, parking, phone calls, etc. Staying at the hospital can get expensive very fast, especially as time is usually needed off from work and bills continue to come in from home.
- o Send a text with nothing but encouragement, and state that you expect nothing back. Sometimes the pressure to respond to

everything is too much; they will respond when they have the energy. Simply receiving a text from a friend who truly cares can make all the difference to a long day. Maybe even set yourself a reminder to remember to text them once a day. While your life is busy and time is flying by, the seconds are ticking by so loudly and slowly for that family.

- Offer to take any other children that they may have for an afternoon of fun. Exhaust them; outside activity if the weather permits. But please, do not load them up on junk food. One parent will be leaving the hospital to care for that child, and they are on auto pilot. A tired child who has had lots of laughter and healthy food takes the pressure off of that parent for the evening, when they are feeling like they have little left to give.
- If they have left their house, take care of their yard for them. Simply send off a text letting them know that their lawn has been mowed, flowers have been watered, or snow has been shovelled.
- Make them some freezer meals. A text, letting them know that when they arrive home you have a few meals to drop off for them, reminds them that people care and that they are not alone.
- If they text you, do your very best to reply in a timely fashion, even though there's a good chance they do not reply to you in the same fashion. Sometimes a mom only has a few minutes outside of those NICU doors and needs someone to simply chat with for five

minutes, before going back to face whatever they are dealing with.

These are only a few ideas. Remember to keep things really practical, simple, and helpful. When their world feels like it is crumbling, having a few friends step up to be the glue will never be forgotten. They may not be able to thank you properly for a few days, weeks, months, or even years depending on the situation; but it is the love that they felt through your acts of service that will never be forgotten. Do what you feel you are able to do for them. Just remember to keep it simple, and make sure that it isn't requiring anything of them. If you need to make all kinds of arrangements and plans that they have to accommodate, maybe you should come up with something else.

I left something unanswered earlier. What is cCMV? It stands for congenital cytomegalovirus. Cytomegalovirus is a very common virus, that is usually harmless in someone with a healthy immune system; it would simply present itself as a cold. I would have had this "cold" in the very early stages of my pregnancy, thus passing it along to the fetus in the very early stages of development, which is why James was born with congenital CMV. CMV is present and spread through bodily fluids. It is a very common virus among preschool and school age children. Once you have had CMV, you carry the antibodies for it, and you are no longer at any risk once you become pregnant. I had never had this before, and therefore it passed on to my baby.

You are probably now wondering how you can prevent your baby from being born with cCMV. There are some very simple things you can do. Things like hand washing seem like common knowledge, but there are so many ways to transmit CMV that we don't think of in our daily lives. And because this is a virus that children are commonly carrying, we need to be so careful when pregnant. Things like a kiss on or near the lips, or sharing a drink with our child can pass this virus on. Things that are so commonly done with young children and seem so harmless.

I don't include this to scare you, only to inform you of what I never knew. I often wonder, if I had known, would James be different today? Could I have done something differently? I will never know, and so I don't let myself stay there.

The best advice I can give is, if you are pregnant, simply ask your Dr. to test your blood to see if you have had CMV before. If you have not, take all those measures, especially when you are around children, even if they are your own. If you have had it before, then pass this information on to the next mamma you talk with. Let's not let this keep happening.

Taking Baby Home
{November 3, 2007}

Having had a few days to process what I had been told, that James would very likely go deaf and blind, but otherwise be totally fine, my heart was rejoicing! I had already done so much reading about congenital cytomegalovirus, and what effects it can have on a child who contracted so early in the pregnancy, so I was feeling so thankful that this was all we were dealing with. I was also blissfully hopeful that neither of those things would even occur.

The next few months are hazy. I lived in a thick fog. This little baby was released to come home, and things were supposed to be as normal as things are when you bring a newborn home. I couldn't reach out to anyone with my true feelings, because I didn't understand my feelings, and others didn't understand the problem like I did. This was my second child, and there was so much more going on than those doctors told me. I knew it in my heart. Everything was so wrong about everything I did with my baby. But if I told people that I knew something was wrong, I got all the typical responses. Oh every child is just so different, this stage is the hardest, you just need to relax honey and things will change naturally, maybe you are doing something wrong, this is completely normal, you probably just need sleep.

Let me be the first to say, I most definitely needed sleep, in mass amounts. James did not sleep. Ever. I don't mean he was up two or three times a night. I mean, for the first two years of his life, he did not sleep for more than an hour consecutively. If he ever slept for an hour and a half it was nothing less than a miracle. Every new mother is exhausted and says her child never sleeps, so no one believed that he only slept for an hour at a time. That was just an assumed exaggeration. But this was no exaggeration. I was a walking zombie, who knew something was so wrong.

James did not eat. I would nurse him for an hour at a time. It felt constant. He would latch on, suck almost nothing, and rip off. And again. And again. And again. I saw a lactation consultant, had a registered nurse come into my home, and went into public health. Nothing helped. I cried, and tried again, and cried, and tried again, and cried. I was devastated. At only two months old we switched him to a bottle. I continued to pump for as long as my milk kept up, but with almost no sleep, that dried up so very quickly. When I made the decision to stop forcing breastfeeding and give him the bottle exclusively, this is the comment I received, "You're just doing this so you can get a babysitter and start going out again." I shattered. That might not seem like a terrible comment, but I shattered. I had tried so hard, I was so devastated. And this came from people who loved me. I am not a person who goes out a lot. I have a few close friends, and one best friend, and my going out usually consists of sitting for hours on end talking with my best friend, sometimes over a meal, or before or after watching a movie cuddled under a blanket. I'm a pretty low key kind of girl. So no, I did not switch my baby to a bottle so that I could ditch him to go out.

Giving him a bottle was not a solution, it was a whole other battle. He couldn't seem to suck from that bottle either. Again I had a nurse come into my home, I went into public health, but none of the positions or new bottles I tried helped. He couldn't get enough. Then he would just stop, like he had no interest. Followed by crying and screaming, until he puked up the very little bit of formula he had actually taken. He sounded raspy all of the time; when he was sitting, lying, eating, making noises, sleeping. I tried every bottle style, every nipple, every level of flow, nothing made a difference. I tried different feeding positions, different bottle temperatures, and different formulas. I tried everything public health suggested, and anything I could find through google.

His body continued to tremor randomly. His whole body would tense up, as if he had been severely startled. Sometimes they were small jerks, sometimes they were violent. Imagine you were falling through the air on your back, you would pull in and get incredibly tense. That is what he would do, and sometimes he would start to cry like he was terrified, like he didn't know where his body was in space. Sometimes he would go from lying peacefully to both arms and legs jerking outwards violently, stiffly. And then he would start to cry. Almost all the time that James did not spend sleeping he spent crying. Not a little newborn coo of a cry. A loud, angry, tired, hungry, scared, terrifying, ear piercing cry. A cry that would make my whole body wince. James would sometimes cry for twenty hours a day, and that is no exaggeration. I don't know how we made it through those days. They were terrible. And still, people thought I was crazy when I shared that I feared something was so wrong.

When James was three months old I called his neonatologist from NICU in Saskatoon. I told them I could not wait until he was six months to come back, I just knew that something was wrong. They booked me in that week and we went back to Saskatoon. I was terrified waiting in that office. He listened to everything I had to say, and then had me lie James down on the examination table in the room. He very thoroughly examined him from head to toe, also doing a neurological examination. He found that the soft spot on James' head had closed already. He explained that meant one of two things. Either it closed in error, and they would have to break his skull to reopen it, so the brain could continue to grow as it needed to. Or, his brain was severely underdeveloped, and would remain so. He said that he would like James to have a CT scan done as soon as possible. He would talk to the nurse and have them call me, and hopefully we would have one done before we even went home. And we did. They called me back about an hour after that appointment, and we were to come back the very next day for a sedated CT scan.

  I was horrified and so relieved at the same time. Someone was listening to me! I was not crazy! James had never been sedated, and his body was so little. I laid awake all that night thinking about this. Would he pull out of it ok? What would the scan show? Finally the morning came, and we were off to the hospital for 7:30am. We went through admitting, and then into the basement of Royal University Hospital, and into the operating room waiting room. Because he was so little they let me come with them, so I followed the nurse down the hall with tiny James in my arms. I got to hold his hand and stroke his forehead on the bed while they put him to sleep. Once he had nodded off I slipped out and into the operating waiting room while the scan was done. Just a short time later I was called from the waiting room to join James in recovery, where I learnt that he came out of anaesthetic horribly. Parents are usually not allowed in recovery, but James' reaction coming out of the anesthetic was far too much for the few nurses in the room to manage. He convulsed, his jaw would lock, he cried and cried, and his whole body was stiff. The convulsions would cause him to cough until he choked, and I would need to roll him onto his side and make sure any liquid that needed to get out could do so. This lasted for about twenty minutes, until his body started to relax, and then we were able to go up to day surgery. Once he could take some liquids we were able to leave. "The neurologist will call within the week once the scan is read if there is anything to report. Have a nice day" the nurse said as we were leaving.

Phew. The scan was done, now I just had to wait that nerve wrecking week for the results. That week came and went, with no phone call. I was so nervous, but anytime I mentioned this to anyone the response was always "no news is good news!" Not for my heart it wasn't. Week two came and went with no news. Now I called our neonatologist. I was informed that our scan wasn't yet read, but obviously there was nothing to worry about or we would have heard already. Week three came and went. Everyone else had written it all off already, everyone except me. I called again, and was told that our scan was maybe not read, or maybe the doctor just hadn't had time to call yet. I less patiently explained that we had now been waiting three weeks and I would like to know something no matter what the results were. Week four. I was losing my mind. All I thought about day and night were these results. And since James and I never slept, it was literally day and night that I had to obsess over this. James was still not eating, not sleeping, crying all day every day, and constantly tremoring.

Finally, the phone rang. My best friend was at my house, and it was lunch time. I left her in the kitchen with my kids and took the phone into my daughte'rs room. It was the head neurologist from Royal University Hospital. Once that introduction happened my heart sank. My world stopped. The head of the department doesn't usually call with phenomenal news. He very gently explained to me that James had extensive brain damage. He had holes throughout his entire brain, many of those holes had calcified, meaning that they had turned to bone. Only part of his brain had even developed, which was why his head was so small. I remember writing what he was saying on a little piece of paper so I wouldn't forget, because my brain had completely shut off. I had tears rolling down my face and my hands were shaking. I can still see that piece of paper perfectly in my mind. My shaky hand had recorded this: the following four things could be expected in his future: severe cerebral palsy, mental retardation, significant motor delays, and seizure disorder. I was absolutely numb. He gave me an appointment date to come in and meet with the neonatologist the next week, and we hung up.

    I just sat there. Really not crying, but tears were still falling off my face. It was like I wasn't even in my body. I came out of my daughter's room, walked back into the kitchen. My best friend wrapped her arms around me. I'm not sure that I spoke much, simply handed over the paper. I don't remember a single other detail from that day. I just completely shut down.

Email Update {Feb 21, 2008}

    First of all, we'd like to say a huge thank you to everyone who has been praying for us through all of this - especially to those of you who told us you were doing so – you never know the impact that has on someone's life until you're in that situation – so thank you!!!!

    For those of you who didn't know that we were going through all these tests we do apologize – it's been a long few months, and our communication hasn't really been the best. There were some concerns originally in NICU with the virus James had – cytomegalovirus – but most of the more severe issues were ruled out at that time. However, in January there were some signs that some things may not have been quite right with the head and brain development.

After a CT that was done at the beginning of February, we now have some answers. His brain has shown many abnormalities, but the full extent won't be fully known for many years. Right now, we know that his brain has many areas that have calcified. He has something referred to as "microcephaly" – meaning that his head is quite small for his size – and will remain small for his size – the brain doesn't fully develop so there is adequate room inside for what is there. There are no issues with the soft spot or skull – as this is the reason that he has almost no soft spot and just has a small head. With the several areas of the brain that are calcified, he has a very high chance of having all or some of the following: delays in development, cerebral palsy, intellectual impairment and seizures. This is all a result of the CMV.

We would greatly appreciate your continued prayers as the next few months will be full of more appointments and tests. James is such a blessing in our lives, and we thank God everyday for bringing him to us. There is a lot of fear going forward as we realize that we are likely not going to be raising the "normal healthy" child that everyone assumes they will be given – but we know that God doesn't bring you to anything that he is not going to carry you through.

Lamentations 3:22-23 says "Because of the Lord's great love we are not consumed, for his compassions never fail. They are new every morning; great is your faithfulness". God knows each and every day what we need of him – and his mercies are new every morning. This is something that has come to mean a lot to me in these last few weeks of waiting

On March 5, 2008, we sat in our neonatologists office, waiting for him to come in and tell us about the results. My husband, James in his little carrier, and I. Dead silence as we waited. Then he came in. He knew why we were there and he immediately got to the point. He had looked at the results and would go over what they meant, and we would be able to meet with the neurologist the following week to ask more questions once we had some time to process what he was telling us. He went over what I was told on the phone. I asked what this meant, his honest opinion, no sugar coating anything. Dr. Givelichian sat down on his stool, wheeled over a little closer to us, and explained that we really couldn't know. However, based on the level of damage he was seeing, his quality of life could be very low, vegetative. There was also a high chance that he would not see very many birthdays. Death was a real possibility. His body was not equipped to fight.

I left that appointment both grateful for such a compassionate doctor, willing to be real with us, and terrified. Terrified at the last statement that he made in that office. My baby could die?

Email Update {March 6, 2008}

Just a quick update on the last few appointments for James. Last week we had an appointment with a pediatric eye specialist – with the CMV he has, the risk of vision problems or blindness is very high. So far, his eyes have developed perfectly, and the nerves from the eyes to the brain are also good. Right now, the brain is not processing what the eyes are seeing properly so he often doesn't pay a lot of attention.

We also had an appointment with his neonatologist yesterday, and here's what the CT shows, and what that means at this time: The white matter (responsible for movement control) and the grey matter (responsible for intellectual functions) in the brain are scattered with cysts, some of which have calcified. All of these cysts are areas of the brain that have not and will not develop. He is behind in meeting his milestones at the age of 4 months – and when an infant is not meeting the basic function milestones, they will be very behind in the higher functions. Based on the medical evidence of what has occurred, there is very little to no chance of James growing up having a "normal" life. Right now, all they can tell us is that he will range anywhere from being mentally slow to not being able to physically move. This was all damage caused in the womb by the CMV. It is not ongoing – the damage is done.... And there is no treatment or surgery to fix anything.

We have an appointment with a pediatric neurologist Wed Mar 12, and James has been placed on the urgent list for an MRI. This MRI is for two reasons: there may be a medication they can put him on to control his involuntary movements if they are being caused by releases from the brain stem. It is also to show more clearly where the majority of the cysts are, and to make a more educated "guess" for his future.

The brain is fully developed by the age of 2 – so we will not know the full effects this will have on him until then.

We thank you for your continued prayers.

On March 12, 2008, we were back at Royal University Hospital in Saskatoon, waiting to see the neurologist. Such a kind nurse came to get us from the noisy pediatric waiting room, where I sat, feeling numb. She asked if we understood why we were there today, and I simply said yes. We were waiting in a small room, until an elderly man entered, so kind and gentle looking. He showed us our results, although it was hard for us to understand what everything meant. He explained that the damage was extensive, but James was really far too young for us to start jumping to any conclusions. We were supposed to have an MRI as soon as possible, but we spent some time talking about the pros and cons to doing that at this time, and he then left the decision up to us.

We could have it now, but it could multiply our fears extensively. And unnecessarily. He was so young that his brain was going to continue to change rapidly anyways. Having the MRI also meant more anesthetic, which he wakes up terribly from. So with all this considered, we decided to put off the MRI.

Again, my heart was so thankful for such a compassionate doctor coming alongside us in this.

Email Update {March 12, 2008}

We just had our appointment with the pediatric neurologist today, and here is the update that we have for you on our precious little James.

We got to actually see the CT scan today, and everything was explained in much more detail to us. We could see the areas of his brain that had excess water, and the many cysts that had calcified. They did a very thorough neurological assessment of James today, and here are the results of that:

James is doing very well over all for a baby with so much brain damage from congenital CMV. He is showing many good signs. Based on the information available right now, the neurologist has said it is very unlikely that James will be as developmentally advanced as Julia, however, that doesn't mean that he won't make great strides and be able to function in society on his own. This neurologist was really amazing...and gave us great hope. We know that there are still soooo many unknowns, and only time will tell.

*they have decided to not do an MRI at this point in time. The MRI would not show anything new – rather – it would just give the neurologist a closer "guess" at what James' future might hold. Because the CT was just done,

and nothing can be done at this point to fix anything, there is no reason to put him under anesthetic again. Also, it could create more fears for us as to his future, and things could change in either direction (I'll explain that below). Rather, they will wait until 12 – 18 months of age unless there is reason to do one sooner. This will show much more as the brain will be much more developed.

*around the age of 1 they will be able to make a close diagnosis as to his future. A baby is born with a brain with many more nerve endings than will ever be used. As they develop, the brain "maps out" the easiest routes to get information where it needs to be, and the rest of the nerve endings eventually die and are never used. Because of the many cysts present, many of those paths have been destroyed. However, the brain is capable at this stage of "remapping" and finding other ways to accomplish things. So, it is a matter of seeing how much of that James is able to do to know how this will affect him in the long run.

*he is doing a lot of good things right now, which can give us a lot of hope. Although his eye contact and general visual awareness is behind where it should be, he is showing a lot of interest in his surroundings, which is a very good sign for a baby with congenital CMV. He also kicks his legs and moves his arms a lot and is able to stretch out when laid on the floor. This shows that his muscles are still loose enough to really be worked on, which could prevent future stiffness.

*based on what they saw of his movements, there is no medication to put him on to control his involuntary movements. We are just to watch these, and video tape them if we are worried about anything that he starts doing. At this point, he has no signs of a seizure disorder, which is common in babies with congenital CMV.

The following is what we are looking at currently as a plan for James' healthcare over the next 6 months – one year:

*regular visits to the Kinsmen Centre for Children in Saskatoon – every 2-3 weeks. These visits include physiotherapy – and they send us home with "homework" to do with James each day. This is critical at this point to ensure he doesn't become more stiff. If he becomes too stiff, his tendons will slowly shorten, causing serious stiffness as he gets older. They also include a visit with a pediatrician, and often a nutritionist/feeding specialist, as stomach problems are common with babies with congenital CMV.

*follow ups with his neonatologist in Saskatoon every 2-3 months.

*At this point, there are no further appointments booked with the neurologist. Everything will go through our pediatrician until further imaging is required in 6 months to 1 year.

*Another hearing exam in May and visual exam in August.

People have been asking how they can be praying for us, so here is how we need people to be praying for James:

*That his brain would be "remapping" in every way possible. The areas of the brain that have calcified are basically areas of bone in the brain – so those parts of the brain have been lost, but the brain has that ability to remap around these areas. It is our prayer that this will be happening constantly.

*That the physiotherapy would be working, and his muscles would be constantly relaxing, and he wouldn't need to have leg braces or be in a wheelchair in the future.

*That he would be able to start relaxing more at night and sleeping longer periods of time. Getting lots of rest is important in giving the brain that time to be "healing" and "remapping". He often has difficulty sleeping because of the involuntary movements.

Again, we would like to thank everyone for all of the prayers, and for the many emails and cards and hugs of encouragement. This really has been a difficult couple of months for us. When someone tells you that your precious baby who looks so perfect to you, has extensive brain damage, it really drops the floor out from under you.

We really had to wrestle with understanding why this happened to our baby, and find a way to continue on in the day to day. John is starting to catch up in his studies again as those got quite behind through all of this – as finding a balance between studies and being there for your family and dealing with his own emotions through this was quite a juggling act.

As we learn more about what is causing many of the abnormalities that we see in James, we are learning better how to handle him and how to make him the most comfortable. We have learnt why he doesn't sleep, and are learning ways to relax his body and help him to sleep. The pieces of the puzzle are finally starting to fit together, and we are starting to make some sense of all this.

We would appreciate your continued prayers for us as a family also as we wait to see what God has in store for this little boy. We have really struggled over the last month with understanding healing and understanding sickness. We have had to open our hearts up to the idea that God could choose to heal this little baby, and we have also had to guard our hearts, and accept that God may not choose to heal this baby. We know that God loves our little James, and that he is holding him in his hands, and we are trusting that God will carry James and our family through whatever the future may hold for us.

Below is a song that I (Dawn) have come to love over the last month. It is Oceans From the Rain by Seventh Day Slumber:

And I'm amazed by You. Cause You're never far away
And all that I've been through, Your love has never changed

You make oceans from the rain
Breathing life into this place
And I will drown inside your love
Until I see your perfect face

And nothing I've acquired means anything at all
Cause you're everything I needed
You're so much more than I deserve

And I thank you Lord
The blood of Jesus can wash your pain away

While yes, it is not ideal for your child to have such brain damage, we are believing that God will "make oceans from the rain". Whether God chooses to heal our baby, and he has that amazing testimony, or he grows up with unknown challenges and uses his kind spirit to show God's love, this little boy is a miracle and a blessing, and will do great things in his life.

With much love,
Dawn, John, Julia and James

The rest of 2008 was spent trying to find a new normal. We had this adorable breathtaking little boy. Who screamed all day every day. My husband was a full time student. My daughter was in preschool. I went back to work part time in the evenings, usually having to call in unable to make my shift because James was sick, and we were sitting in a clinic, or an emergency room, or waiting for a prescription.

2008 was filled with pneumonia and bronchitis, antibiotics and nebulizers for James. Puke and coughing fits and crying for hours and hours on end. He was so hungry, but he wasn't strong enough to eat, and what I did get into him he threw up. He aspirated everything he ate, bringing on the chest infections, leading to the coughing, and the puking; the cycle went on and on and on.

    I spent night after night rocking him in the living room. We would both fall asleep for an hour here and there. Then his tiny body would jerk him awake, and he would cry. And I would cry. And he would scream. And I would try unsuccessfully to feed him. Followed by walking him, trying desperately to get the screaming to stop, until hours later when we both passed out for another hour.

    Imagine your worst night dealing with colic. Now do that every single night for two years. Julia was colicky very badly for about three weeks when she was one month old, and I thought I was going to die then! In the dark it felt like hell. In the morning it felt like hell. Now throw in a toddler who wants to play and no family near enough to help. Friends who were terrified of your screaming baby. And everyone else who knew what we were going through, but stayed far enough away so that they wouldn't be uncomfortable.

    I remember talking with a neighbour in the driveway one day, and they were saying that they still hadn't met James! I explained to them that really we rarely ever left the house, and told them why. She lightheartedly said it couldn't possibly be that bad, and invited themselves over for coffee that night – they would bring the dessert, we would catch up on our lives, and she could hold James! I warned her that he would likely scream through the whole ordeal, but she didn't think that was likely. So after supper, her and her husband came over for dessert and coffee, and we all sat in the living room. And guess what? James was screaming when they walked in the door. James screamed the entire time they were there. James screamed when she tried to hold him, rock him, walk him, sing to him and play with him. And, James was still crying when they left. She looked at me a few times during the evening with eyes saying "I am just so sorry." She sat on the floor with me, and wanted to hear about everything we had tried, and everything we had learnt.

Not surprisingly, another dessert date did not happen. It was far too much for people to handle. And once they had seen it, people no longer knew how to interact with me. Once they had seen it there was no ignoring it or playing ignorant to the reality that this adorable baby screamed and cried all day.

Email Update {August 14, 2008}

We have been receiving a lot of inquires lately as to how James is doing, so I've decided to send out an update.

First of all, thank you again to those of you who have kept our family in your prayers. It is so encouraging to hear from someone that they are still praying for you through this... so thank you from the bottom of our hearts.

James is now almost 10 months old, and still functioning physically at about a 4 month level. He doesn't roll over, and is no where near being able to sit. His hand coordination is slowly getting better – he now brings his hands to his mouth, and is able to touch his knees (both really great milestones!!). Mentally, James is very alert and responsive!!

We have now stopped receiving treatment at the Kinsmen every 2 weeks in Saskatoon. We just received the call today that they will be able to do his Physiotherapy and Occupational Therapy right in Moose Jaw – what an answer to prayer!! I have also found a registered physiotherapist right here in Caronport who has her own practice now, who started her career working with developmentally delayed babies – so we will also be bringing James to her once a week starting in the fall.

We will be going to Saskatoon at the beginning of September for an appointment with his neonatologist, and an eye appointment. At the end of September we will be back again for hearing tests – because of his age, they will be putting him under anesthetic to do these....which we aren't crazy about – but they have a pediatric ENT, and registered nurse from pediatrics, the senior audiologist, and the anesthetist all booked for 4 hours to do these tests and will all be in the room the whole time with him – so he will be in good hands!

He will be followed up by a neurologist in Regina in January. Likely, they won't do an MRI until next fall, to give us the best possible "guess" at what the future will look like for us.

He has started choking a lot during the day, and often results in him bringing up everything from his stomach... We're not sure if this is the start of stomach problems, which we have been told from the beginning can become severe, or merely just a phase.

John will be returning to school full time in a few weeks, and I will be going back to work. Julia will be starting preschool in September, every Tuesday and Thursday morning – she is very excited about this!

We would appreciate your continued prayers as this still breaks our hearts every single day. And at the same time, we couldn't have asked for a bigger blessing in our lives.

What Might Have Been
{December 2008}

In our small little village, the college puts on a Christmas musical every year, and the night of the musical, I was working a shift in the local coffee shop. There were two of us working, as it was very busy with all the extra people in for the musical. The night was going wonderfully, sometimes anything felt like a step up from walking a screaming, puking baby for endless hours with no break in sight! That was, until I started to experience abdominal pain. I tried to wait it out, but it wouldn't leave. Instead, it was getting considerably worse, so bad that I could hardly stand anymore. I left to quickly use the washroom. It wasn't quick.

I have barely ever even talked about this to anyone, let alone written down the details. It was months before I even told my husband. Over a year before I told anyone else.

When I got into that stall I locked the cold metal door, pulled down my pants, and sat down. Then I noticed the blood in my underwear, and soaked through just barely to my pants. Thankfully they were black so it really wasn't noticeable. I could hear something falling into the toilet, but it wasn't voluntary. I can still hear it so clearly; I was so confused. I stood for a moment, to see clots. Clots in the toilet, clots now falling to the floor, clinging like sticky tentacles to my legs. Thick strings of blood and mucous, so much pain, and now tears. I was pregnant. I had missed a cycle, several weeks prior, but that was not unusual for me; I thought nothing of it, until right now. That was me losing my baby. My baby that I never knew I was even carrying, but I immediately loved. And mourned. In a bathroom stall of a gas station, alone, on shift. How do your mourn something that you never even knew you had? I was in there for an hour, and all I could do was cry, and flush the toilet in between people coming and going. My co-worker came to check on me once, and I said I'd be out soon.

After an hour, I went out to finish the last hour of my shift. I served a never ending line up of people their lattes and espressos and hot chocolates, numbly, and closed up for the night. I walked home through my quiet little town at midnight and cried the whole way. I was crying so much that I just crawled onto the couch for the night when I got home, until of course, James woke crying.

I didn't tell a soul. James was only fourteen months old, and I knew what people would say. I knew I couldn't handle what they would have to say. "It's for the best;" "you already have your hands full anyways;" "it could have ended up just like James;" "this was probably a blessing." So I told nobody. And women never used to talk about this. So many people have been in this exact spot, but nobody knew. I mentioned it to my husband months later, I think just in casual conversation. Nothing really ever came of it; I think we just had too much going on, and I mentioned it too casually. And really, unless you are a woman who has been through this, how can you understand it? It sounds petty. It sounds like over dramatized grief, doesn't it? Like maybe you need a little more drama in your life so you can stop obsessing over something that really never even was? Yet, it was. It was a life. I believe that a life begins at conception. And I believe that one day I will meet that little treasure that I never had the privilege of holding. I still get that pain in my heart when I see a new born baby. When I hear another mother tell her story of loss. I don't think that part of your heart ever really moves on.

I saw my doctor after, we discussed what happened, and he examined me. Nothing further was required medically, my body had done its job.

One day a year later, a friend met me after work to walk home with me. She shared through tears that she had just lost a pregnancy, and that was the first time I shared just a little from my own story. It felt so good to cry with someone. I have found the value in learning to hurt with people. Learning to share my hurt, knowing that vulnerability opens the door for healing.

This is still a hurt that I carry in my heart, but do not know how to talk about. I still yearn for that baby; that baby that I never held in my arms, kissed on the forehead, lowered softly into bed for the night. It is something that only a mother who has lost an unborn child can fully understand. It is a piece of your heart that you give away forever.

The year was not without its victories! James became more alert, more tuned into his surroundings. He was recognizing family in between visits, something we didn't know if he would be able to do. My parents came to stay with both children in November, and the husband and I went to Banff for two nights to recharge and relax. And that little boy, who I had been working so so hard with every single day, decided to roll over for the very first time with grandma! What a little stinker! I was walking in a toy store in Banff when my mom called to tell me, and I remember crying! Partly because I was so happy for this milestone! And partly because after all of my hard work I was not there for this. This was not a regular thing until late 2009, but it did happen once. It only happened once every few weeks afterward, but it was a huge step that all his therapists were so pleased to know was happening, even though he refused to show them his new skill!

Overall, we survived 2008. My heart survived 2008. Endured. Enduring does not signal a win or a victory. I held on to what I could every day to get through. I was a complete ugly terrifying mess in my mind. But my heart remained soft and hopeful. Hopeful that one day we would sleep. And laugh. And sleep again ☺

{2009}

James is now just over two years old, and this year brought out more confidence and fight in me. This was the year I fought for a feeding tube for James. It had been on my mind for quite some time, but it terrified anyone that I brought it up to. After all, a feeding tube is classified as life support. It was admitting defeat, taking the easy road, succumbing to the disability. But it wasn't! It would give him a fighting chance! It would let his lungs breathe and his stomach handle the food! It was time to fight.

You will read more about this battle later on, but James got his first Mic-key button g-tube in November of 2009. Finally, after a whole year of continuous, over lapping bouts with bronchitis and pneumonia, caused by aspiration. And from that day on we had an IV pole and feeding pump set up beside the table., and were serenaded by the "click, click, click" of that pump at every meal time. Food now safely entered his stomach, not his lungs; and his lungs were able to heal finally. He was no longer dehydrated, and very slowly our lives started to change from here on out.

James began to sleep for two to three hours at a time after the surgery. Which meant I began to sleep for two to three hours at a time!

As a comparison, here is a look at a typical night from October 2007 – September 2009 (0-23 months of age):

- 8:00 pm – medication, snack and pyjamas
- 8:30 pm – rock James to sleep
- 9:00 pm – lie James in his crib and try to sneak out of his room. Make it half way to the door when he wakes and begins screaming. Back to the rocking chair in the living room
- 10:00 pm – Still rocking James. His body relaxes, then convulses violently waking him, he cries for half an hour, and falls back asleep.
- 11:00 pm – try again to put James into bed. Stand up, and he wakes. Sit back down and begin to rock him. He is now screaming again, and John is going to bed, as he has college classes in the morning.
- 12:00 am – James is still jerking awake. I fall asleep holding him, until a jerk is so violent that it wakes us both. He is screaming, and I begin walking him in circles in the living room, hoping that his screaming does not wake his dad or his sister.
- 1:00 am – I am exhausted from walking him in tiny circles. He is exhausted, but still screaming. I am crying, and I lay him down to use the bathroom, where I cry, from exhaustion and frustration. I hurry back to pick him up, and hope that my calm body language will transfer to him. It doesn't. He is stiff and rigid and screaming as though he is in so much pain that nothing can help.

- 2:00 am – We both drift into a light sleep in the rocking chair, maybe even for an hour. Until his tiny arms and legs all jerk outward, as if falling from the sky, and he is again screaming. I can barely keep my eyes open, so I lift his tiny tight body and we begin walking again. I sing to him, talk to him, pray for him, pray with him, cry out for help. James is still screaming.
- 3:00 am – I cannot do it any longer. I lie him in his crib, still screaming, and I lie on the floor beside him, where I pass out. I wake up within moments, to his shrills and scoop him back up. He calms at my touch, but only for moments. That pained cry returns almost immediately.
- 4:00 am – we are back in the rocking chair in the living room. Will it ever end? I wrap him tightly and at some point we both fall back to sleep. He violently jerks several more times, waking us both, beginning the cycle of screaming all over again. We get a few chunks of half hour sleep before Julia wakes between 6:00am and 7:00am.

Now to compare that schedule, when things began to change after he received his feeding tube.

- 8:00 pm – medication, snack and pyjamas.
- 8:30 pm – rock James to sleep
- 9:00 pm – Attempt to put James into bed. Carry him to his room, lie him in bed (he now has a single bed with a railing), and his body jerks awake as soon as he isn't being held tightly. Return to the rocking chair in the living room.

- 10:00 pm – Still rocking James. His body jerks awake, the crying begins, and we continue to rock. After about a half an hour he begins to settle.
- 11:00 pm – Try again to get James into bed. This time I get him into bed, and begin walking away. He jerks awake moments later and the crying starts. I take him out of bed and we return to the rocking chair. We both fall asleep with him tightly bundled in my arms.
- 2:00 am – We wake up in the chair. John has turned off all the lights and has long gone to bed. James and I are still in the rocking chair with the tv on. I take him back to bed, and his body startles as I lie him down, and the crying instantly begins again. I leave, turn off the television, and return to his bed. This time I simply crawl into his bed, hold him tightly, and we both fall back asleep, usually with me in tears, and we sleep until the morning. Sometimes he wakes a few times in there, and sometimes we sleep straight until about 6:00 am.

You will notice that his body jerks him awake often, yet we did not swaddle him tightly. The reason? Because when his body jerks, his arms fly up, and he takes the biggest breath you can imagine. Like someone with sleep apnea would do after stopping breathing. Except James does not have sleep apnea (we had him tested). This was just what his body did and if we swaddled him with his arms trapped in the swaddle, we would take away his ability to get his arms up and get in that deep breath that he needed.

You will also notice that when he cries, I am there. There are several reasons for that – many of which most people never fully understand. Why not sleep train him? He needs to cry to learn to self soothe. He will learn you just need to give him more time. He needs to cry longer. Nope. Nope. And NO! This was not my first rodeo! I tried sleep training with him. I did it with Julia, so why can't I do it with James? This wasn't a cry for mom. It was a cry like his body hurt. Like something was happening that we couldn't figure out. Maybe something was happening in his brain? Nobody knew. Medication didn't help. Pain killers didn't help. Melatonin didn't help. Sleep medication did not help. Letting him cry it out did not help. Letting him cry without a body next to him never worked. Letting him cry until he choked, and puked, was all that was ever accomplished. And then the pained cry started all over, worse than it began, and no sleep happened for the rest of the night.

His body needed pressure. But it could not be a tight swaddle, or a weighted blanket. He was not strong enough to move either on his own in the case that he needed to throw those arms up to take that breath that he needed, which was constant. He couldn't roll when he started to choke; he needed me there to instantly do that for him. Without my body against his, and my arms holding him tightly, his rigid little body could not relax enough to fall asleep. And once he was asleep, he needed that pressure to stay asleep. Once I fell asleep and my wrap on him loosened, his jerks would wake him and we would start all over again.

The change between those two sleep schedules really is huge!! While you may be reading that thinking – those are both terrible! The second one, after his surgery, was a life changing thing for me. A small chunk of sleep every night was amazing! Granted, I had a snoring, jerking, violent, loud little boy beside me almost every night, so my sleep was far from deep. But it was sleep! And I would take anything I could get!

The fog began to lift. It really took years to lift, to see and feel clearly again, but the process started right here with that g-tube. If others wanted to see James as being on life support, I decided not to care! This was about his quality of life, and his quality of life was vastly improving before our eyes.

We didn't have any adaptive chairs for James in our home. We were given a corner seat, which he used once in a while, but hated. We were offered one other chair; it was metal, sat on the floor, and looked like something out of an institution. We have always tried to keep things very homey for him, keeping harsh medical equipment out of the picture. And this chair was a no brainer for us; it was not coming home! We bought a peg perego high chair, and because of the tilt in space feature, it worked perfectly for in the home! Friends fund raised for us, and we purchased a special tomato pushchair with some inserts for more support, and it was perfect for what he needed. We brought it with us into the Kinsmen Children's Centre in Saskatoon when we went, and the therapists absolutely loved it, and made sure he was supported properly in there for us. It was far better than what they were able to offer us at the time.

Early Childhood Intervention came into our home twice a month and we worked on goals which I would be able to lay out. They would lend us wedges and rolls for me to be able to do therapy at home, and any toys that he seemed interested in they would lend to us until he became uninterested in them. They were my support when dealing with so many different health professionals and therapists. They gave us information on programs that could help us. Our worker cared and we became friends. She had a daughter with cerebral palsy who had passed away when she was very young, and so she connected with James. She knew my struggles as a mom, I could tell her about my hard days. I didn't have to hide when my eyes welled up with tears as we talked through different scenarios and situations.

James got his first pair of AFO's this year – ankle foot orthosis. Tiny itty bitty little plastic splints to keep his feet and ankles at the proper angle to his little legs, which were still somewhat chubby at this point! Little hard blue AFO's decorated with dinosaurs. He was so very tiny to be sitting in the orthotics office, having casts made from the knees down, but it was so adorable. He never minded them – I don't think he really knew they were there. And he only needed to wear them for about thirty minutes a day at this point. I probably spent more time taking them out to show everyone because they were so cute than I did actually putting them on him.

{2010}

In 2010 James changed so much. He was now a chubby little three year old baby. He was able to roll, but mostly got around by lying on his back and pushing with his right leg. His concentration was getting longer and he enjoyed playing with toys for short periods of time.

He had a cat scan done this year, which really showed us the miracle that he was. I will go into detail about this amazing event a little later on.

In February our ECIP worker brought up the subject of school, and asked if we would like to choose inclusion and have him attend the same school where Julia would be starting kindergarten in the fall, or if we would like to know more about the school in Moose Jaw. It was a ten minute drive away, where they had a program all set up for developmentally challenged children. School?? To be honest, I was pretty sure this lady was losing her mind! At this time James was barely two and a half years old!

After I spent some time looking at her like she had possibly escaped from some kind of an institution, she realized I had no idea why she was telling me any of this! Apparently, when you have a child as delayed physically and mentally as James was, they start full time school at the age of three. I had kind of figured it would be the other way around and he would start school much later than "normal" children. You think dropping your child off for the first half day of Kindergarten at age five is hard? I was supposed to let my baby James, who was so very tiny, and completely non verbal, just go to school without me?! I'm still thinking this lady is absolutely nuts at this point!

Well, we ended up deciding against full inclusion, a decision every family has to make based on their child's individual needs. James was so little, and so different, but he just wanted to be included in everything! Our small community school was just not equipped to handle his needs. There would be no one to tube feed him while at school. And he would likely be assigned an aide, and would spend most of his time in a corner in the classroom, or removed from the classroom because his noises would be too distracting for everyone else. We didn't want him to be segregated. We didn't want his differences to seem so evident.

We chose the school that was already set up for him. It was a catholic elementary school with one wing labelled as the development centre. They had their own entrance into the school, one teacher (which quickly changed to two teachers), about ten educational assistants, and two nurses. They also had physical therapists who came in to assess equipment being used and to set up daily therapy routines for the nurses to do with the children. Speech language and behavioral therapists also regularly visited. Children were often integrated into the appropriate classroom within the school for half an hour up to half a day each day, depending on their needs. They had wheelchair buses to take the children to and from school, and often went on outings such as bowling, swimming, and Mass.

I would love to tell you the James loved school and did so well in this transition, but he didn't! It was awful! You know the book entitled "Alexander and the Terrible, Horrible, No Good, Very Bad Day", the 2010-2011 school year for James could have been called "James and the Terrible, Horrible, No Good, Very Bad First Year of School". No kidding! He went from full time down to two hours a day. And he would come home at the end of those two hours with no voice, from crying all morning at school. I actually pulled him out of school for a month mid October, because my concerns were not being properly addressed by his teacher, and I was not going to start James' schooling off being bullied into things that I did not agree with. So I pulled him, and stated that once we worked out a few things I would bring him back.

Mid November James returned to school, and we stuck to 9-11am until Christmas. He still cried every day, but it was becoming slightly less. After Christmas we moved to half days and I picked him up at noon. Around March we extended it until 1pm, and for the month of June he went full days, in preparation for the next year.

It was really hard to send him to school so young. You always worry about your children when you send them off, but when they are unable to talk to you, tell you how people are treating them, how they feel, it is so much harder.

I learnt to trust my instinct. If something wasn't right with him I would call the school, until I could figure out what it was. I also dropped in regularly and without notice. I wanted to know that he was always safe and being taken care of properly. At first this was not an issue. At some point, signs went up that you needed to ring a bell in the entrance when you arrived and you would be let in, however I never abided by this. If there was nothing to hide then I saw no issue with simply dropping in once a month to see how things were going. No one ever said anything to me so I continued to do so!

By the end of this year at school James was starting to have a relationship with a few of the aides and trust was being built. He even had a few days where he didn't cry at all! Change was so hard for him. Because of his many health issues up until this point, he was used to always having mom with him. So this adjustment was so huge, and so hard, but slowly and with time, he was adjusting.

Almost no progress was made at school as far as skill development, but very small social steps had been taken. He was still very unsure about every environment that did not include me, and crying fits were still his chosen way to communicate this. But after a year of hard work, he was beginning to recognize patterns and schedules within the day that offered him some sense of safety. He looked forward to circle time each morning, when all of the staff and students gathered in one room for singing and attendance.

Things really started looking up, I could see light amidst all the dark. Hope was returning that I would slowly come out of my fog. And somehow, this is when I would say that my battle with depression intensified.

Depression

I have struggled with anxiety and depression for a lot of my adult life, but both have intensified since the birth of James. To say that they have intensified is likely not the truth. Coming through the years of almost no sleep, with the many fears and struggles along the way, I more likely didn't have the time to know myself well enough, and to be able to healthily work through these things.

As I write this, James will be turning seven this month. We made it to seven! And I now understand myself well enough to know my warning signs, and to know exactly what my body needs to counter it. I start to think only of myself and how situations are affecting me. I stop sleeping, the tears come all too easily. It feels as if the wind has been knocked out of me quite literally, it is a struggle to breathe. Everything in my day feels as though it is screaming at me, not allowing a second of silence. I'm questioning every decision I make, losing that trust that I usually have in myself. I am fighting all day long with myself. And it doesn't end when I go to bed; the voices become louder. It's exhausting and overwhelming.

This happened just last week. Three days of this before I finally said to myself, I'm letting this win. I know exactly what is happening and I have to fight.

And I fought. I made myself lie down every afternoon, whether I slept or not. If I couldn't come up with a healthy solution to a problem, the answer was to take a nap. I ate vegetables and protein. Red peppers, avocado, chick peas, beans, tomatoes, spinach; these all seem to balance me out. I exercised. Like exercised until I was a disgusting sweaty mess exercised. I ran out my voices and fears on the treadmill in our basement to loud music. I began taking iron and vitamin b. I keep these on hand because I know that these are the two things that my body regularly dips extremely low on, and I need to get these balanced before I will start to feel differently. I stay away from all processed foods. I maintain the cleanliness in our home, but I do not worry about the extras. I take extra time to sit and watch a movie and cuddle with my children. I lie in bed and talk on the phone with my best friend once the kids are in bed. And while this all sounds lovely and cushy, every single second of this is torture. I do all of these things against the loudness in my head. I am fighting the whole entire day. I am often still fighting through the night. But slowly things start to change. Everything slowly becomes balanced, and everything relaxes. The fight leaves.

This battle hasn't always been this manageable for me. I never used to recognize it. I didn't know that my iron and vitamin b were triggers. I didn't know when it was starting, and to pay attention to every single thing that I was putting in my body and doing with my body. How is that even possible when you are living on two hours of sleep a day, listening to blood chilling screaming all day every day, and trying to sort out the life of your child? It isn't.

The best advice I can offer is to allow yourself grace. Allow yourself to feel it. And tell at the very least one person your honest raw heart. Let someone know how badly you are struggling. They can't fix you. And if you are expecting that, then you may be setting up a relationship failure.

I remember one night, when James was about twelve months old. We knew about the cCMV and the intense brain damage, but he hadn't yet been officially diagnosed with cerebral palsy. He had been screaming for days. Literally. I laid him in his crib and I fell to the floor. And right there I begged God, out loud, in frantic sobs, to please take James home. This life was so unfair for him, and I was too broken to do this well. Please God, take my baby home. Let him be healthy in heaven. Why do you continue to torture my baby? Please take him. Set his body free.

It rips my heart out to even write these words. What kind of mother pleads with God to let her child die? What kind of mother throws in the towel like that? I remember my pain in that moment. Excruciating physical pain from the exhaustion. Screaming in my head that would not stop. The need for it to all stop.

James continued to scream. And I laid on his floor beside the crib and sobbed and sobbed. I cried until I passed out. When I woke up he was still screaming. I stood up and lifted his frail little body out of his crib and rocked him. He would settle and melt into me, until his body violently jerked, and the screams would start all over again. We did this all night.

In moments such as those, I was too tired to recognize depression and anxiety. I felt trapped, and angry, and alone, with no sign of hope. Or help. Those days are long gone. And all I truly remember of them is the feeling of being tortured, almost like drowning. Have you ever had one of those dreams where something bad is happening to you, but when you try to scream nothing comes out? You keep trying, but no sound ever comes out. That is what I remember feeling. Not knowing how to reach out, what to say, how to balance the crazy enough to let someone in. It was torture. I was trapped in my own personal hell. Not only was I dealing with the screams coming from my baby that I could not stop, the screams on the inside were even worse, and I couldn't get away from them.

I didn't get through these times well. I didn't confide in anyone, no one knew the inner torture that was far worse than everything I was dealing with on the outside. Anyone who has dealt with depression or anxiety will agree that talking to only yourself in the midst of it is one of the worst things you can do. It's like a hamster running on a wheel, there will never be an out. You will never find a new rationale. You will never be able to reason with those inner voices alone. All I wanted to do was stop the loudness that was taking over my mind.

Now, my struggle lies more in finding purpose in my life. The world sees success as money, recognition, worldly possessions. And I have contentedly traded all of these to make James' life all that it can be, which I wouldn't trade for the world! However, that self doubt creeps in all too often. You've accomplished nothing with your life. You can't do anything. You can't go there, your clothes aren't good enough. You can't be seen there, you haven't worked out enough. The difference these days, is I only drown for a day or two, and then I recognize the pain for what it is. And I know what I am needing to do to fight it.

Very few people know that I struggle with depression, because again, we don't talk about our weaknesses. We want people to think that we are strong, to admire us, to want to be with us. But we forget that our hearts are all the same. We are all struggling with something, we are all hurting in some way. We are all walking a slightly different path than that one we dreamed of while sipping on tea from mini porcelain pink rose teacups and eating tiny oreos. When we are vulnerable enough to share with other, even if the stories are completely different, the hurt feels manageable. We all feel less alone, more capable of fighting through the hopelessness. I am learning to be more honest, but I struggle in this area. I am able to reach out to people who I know are also struggling with depression or anxiety, but I struggle to be the first one to share. And I have rarely shared with someone who does not struggle. It makes me feel like I am less, like I am weaker. I worry that if you know that I have anxiety attacks, that you will assume that is what is happening when you don't agree with my emotional response to a situation. I worry that if you know that I struggle with depression that you will simply assume that is what is going on when I share my hurts or fears in my lonely walk with James. I worry that if you know, you will hold back from sharing your struggles with me, thinking that I have too much going on to be able to step into your world authentically. I worry that you will analyze my past, and think that you see where my depression or anxiety were affecting me, when in reality, that was merely where you saw an honest glimpse at my reality.

James is seven, almost eight now, and my anxiety has the ability to rip through me the way a fire can take over a house in seconds. I have taken James into my bed with me for the last three nights now, because he is going through one of his cycles where his body cannot relax enough to allow him to sleep. And after several hours of carrying his long sleeping body from the couch to his bed, lying him down, and his body waking him, and having to carry him back to the couch, my body is too tired to continue. And so I have taken him to bed with me. Sometimes he is able to fall into a deep sleep beside me and we both sleep peacefully. Other nights he pulls my hair, hits me, yells at me, all while his body jerks, he gasps for air, and he continually wakes up choking all night long. My anxiety is triggered by lack of sleep, but there isn't a lot that I can do to stay away from this cycle. I simply have to learn to live the best that I can through it.

Anxiety feels like someone has their hands wrapped around your heart, and they are very literally trying to squeeze the life out of you. It is work to breathe, my chest feels heavy, I have to breathe slowly and consciously, feeling the breath reach the very bottom of my lungs. And then remember to do it all over again once I have exhaled. It feels as though an elephant is sitting on my chest, and with each breath I have to move that beast up and down. When I am anxious, I cannot think past the day. I cannot think about the tasks I need to do tomorrow, or next week. If I do, I cancel all of those plans. It all piles up in my mind and I cannot compartmentalize it, so I clear it all out, cancel everything so that I can breathe. It isn't rational, but rational isn't exactly the definition of anxiety!

I can't get the big picture when I am anxious. I can't see that everything with James happens in cycles, it just feels as though it will go on forever. Whether we are talking about his sleeping patterns, his stiffness, vomiting, or the crying spells. I may remember that he operates in cycles, and my head may know that he cannot cry forever, but my reality does not accept it. All I hear is the full day, or two, or three, of crying and yelling. All I feel is the week of sleepless nights that I am trying to operate through. All I see is all my hard work with feeding going down the drain when he pukes multiple times every day for days on end.

I can't step away from the scene and prioritize and tackle. Normally, if James pukes, and it is on him, the carpet, and me, I can quickly make a plan of attack, and have everyone and everything cleaned up within minutes, and it doesn't disrupt the day. If my anxiety is raging, that is definitely not the case. Talk about tunnel vision and deer in the headlights. I can see it all, but how am I supposed to do all of this, on top of everything else, and it is just going to happen again. The cleanup takes much longer, and there is much less joy at the end of it all.

How am I dealing with it these days? Still mostly alone. I will talk about it occasionally, but it's still pretty rare. Really I just breathe through it. Find some pressure. A heavy blanket, or lying on my stomach for a while. If my husband is home, I like to sneak on his heavy bullet proof vest. It is the ultimate anxiety hug. And try to zoom out a little from the present chaos. I try not to let myself make decisions for any day other than the day that I am dealing with – or else I will cancel everything in sight on that calendar!

Time away, for only me, quiets my mind and allows me to refocus. Mat Kearney. Ships in the Night. I'm not sure what it is about this song, but I can smell rain in the air when I hear this song. Feel the cool Saskatchewan prairie breeze in my hair. I get a rush of adrenaline. I feel refreshed.

The summer after my cancer surgery I started biking on the grid roads around the small village where we lived. I was biking thirty to fifty kilometers a day. I biked on hot days, windy days, and rainy days. On the rainy days I would just avoid the dirt roads, because in Saskatchewan those roads are clay and I had to walk my bike two kilometers in the field beside that clay road one time when I risked it! Of all those memories, the feeling of being free, alone, quiet, and the smell of rain in the cool air is what stuck with me. And this album was my favorite to bike to, this song in particular.

We all need something to escape to. My escape is always changing, as my freedom is always changing. Now that we have moved and my husband is away working or sleeping the majority of the time, I don't get away like I used to. I have started writing. Some of it I keep, some of it I don't. Sometimes I write something fun just because it's fun, and calming. Sometimes I sneak away for a twenty minute bubble bath. If it is nice and the kids are in school, I walk for hours, or bike, or just sit in the sun.

I Don't Even Know My Own Son

I so often stop and just look at James, and feel so deeply sad. I feel this sadness for two reasons; because he must feel so trapped, imprisoned within his own body. And the second, because he must feel unknown.

Can you imagine a life where you understood all that was happening around you, and yet you had no way to respond in a way that everyone else understood? Can you even begin to fathom how it would feel to understand your surroundings and their happenings, and to also understand that your reaction and response to those surroundings would not be understood by those around you? To want to run, but not even be able to stand? To smell steak, to know that everyone else is carried away to a little bit of heaven as they eat, and yet know that you cannot chew?

He must feel confined in school, coming into the gymnasium for assembly, seeing all the kids his age laughing and sitting in rows on the floor, while he is stuck at the back, with the special needs class, that many pretend do not even exist. We take him swimming with us every time we go, but he always has to get out early. His body becomes so cold, and you can only put that skinny little body in the hot tub for so long before you have to take him out of there also. And then he disappears to the change room, while his sister and whoever else came along is still laughing and splashing in the water.

Our doctor talked to us years ago about watching for signs of depression and anxiety in James. He has always displayed signs of anxiety, as he relies so heavily on me for everything, so seeing me walk away caused deep anxiety. This seems to be getting better naturally as he gets older. But the depression. If I could spend one day inside his beautiful mind, hearing what he is thinking, feeling, seeing, wanting, needing, yearning for. How long can someone feel trapped and not feel a form of depression? How long can our love shelter him? The love of a family can change their world, and it has done miracles for James, but does that run out? Does there come a point where love alone is no longer enough? Do the disappointments start lingering, lasting?

Does James feel unknown? I wonder this, because I feel like I have never truly known him, and I may never truly know him, despite the fact that I know this little boy deeper than anyone else on this side of heaven. In heaven, I will know him as God created him to be.

So often we hear, "God created him like this to teach us all something." No. James was not made to be disabled to teach you how to love, or be thankful, or anything else you may come up with. James was created to be a boy who talks, walks, yells, articulates, creates, explores, imagines, designs, loves, and I could go on forever. James was created with a purpose. And yes, while he is carrying out a purpose on this earth, a purpose far greater than mine most likely, and a purpose that reaches so much farther than I could possible imagine, he is not as he was originally created to be.

I wonder, would he be loud, his imaginings making me pull out my hair some days? Would he be sweet, taking care of mommy when I was sick? How would his voice sound? How would his voice sound saying, "I love you." Would he be strong willed like his sister, always having an opinion about everything? Or would he be quiet? Would he be soft hearted and sensitive, or rough and energetic?

And while yes, I know James' traits, and I love each one of them, I know he would be so different if he wasn't so trapped. If he could have the freedom that he craves, he would be developing and learning, and his character would change to some degree. I can say what I think his character is now, and it would be fairly close, but I would be so wrong on so many things I am sure.

I know so many who are care givers to their children struggle with this. We have never known our child any other way, and we love them for who they are, at every stage. And we treasure every stage that we get to hold them for. But we wonder who they would be if things had been different. Who they could become. What they would do in this world. We worry that one day they will start to understand how trapped they are. We worry that they will feel depression, and not be able to tell us. And while we may see it happen, even if we do catch it and recognize it for what it is, we still do not have a way in to be able to help them beyond medication. We worry that one day our love for them and between us and them will no longer get us in deep enough to make the difference that we desperately want to make.

I was watching a show called "Once Upon a Time" with my best friend one day, and Pinocchio was in this particular scene. Pinocchio was coming to life, transforming from wood to a young boy, right in front of his father. And all I could think was, what would it feel like to have James be able to stand up, run into my arms, talk to me, and control his own body.

We love them exactly where they are at. We learn from their smiles and joy and laughter. We break with their screams and tears and tight bodies and limitations. And we long to know them , on a level that we take so for granted with our unaffected children.

Failing

Today I feel as though I have failed, am failing, and I wish that this was a new feeling. July 2015. This afternoon I spent the afternoon cooking up a new four meal batch of whole food blenderized formula. Then I spent thirty minutes fighting to get it into James' tube. I had to disconnect his extension, twice, to completely unclog it. The medicine port burst open three times, spewing formula all over my face, body and carpet. The syringe slipped out of the extension twice, releasing a river of formula and stomach contents onto my lap and the floor. And I dumped a total of ten feeds down the drain.

So for supper today, orally, he ate 1/3 cup of vegetable soup, two cottage cheese perogies with sour cream, and a vanilla pudding. By tube he only got maybe 50 calories, followed by a half cup of whole milk and water. Not a total write off for a normal seven year old child. But James burns atleast twice the amount of calories as an active child his age.

Tonight my heart hurts, aches. I know, big deal, I had to dump some food. But food is such a stress, such a struggle. I just want so badly for him to enjoy food the way that we do. That will never fully happen, so I need to find my peace with how we need to do things. I put so much time into his nutrition, planning his meals orally, and by tube, to optimize the nutrients, fibre, protein, fat and calories that he is getting. But it is just impossible to get right. This is something that seems so basic, so natural. But every pound is such a struggle.

Failure is something that I rarely talk about, but I feel it almost every day. Everywhere I go is a reminder that I'm not doing enough, that I cannot do enough. Every conversation is a reminder of that. Don't get me wrong – I don't wallow in it! Rarely do I sit and let it consume me, as I did this evening. But it is lurking in the back of my mind consistently.

I listen to friends talk about what their children did today. What they did yesterday. Their grand plans as a family for summer holidays. James gets out far more than the average child with his level of disability. I don't let what he cannot do stop us from doing things! I simply carry him, push him, make accommodations for him. But I don't fit into these conversations very well. And I feel failure.

I work tirelessly to keep my house clean for him, because he rolls around it. And still, I get comments on how unclean I am. I make all the accommodations I can to keep up to "normal" life with friends and family, but I am still seen as pulling away because of the limitations that stay. We cannot keep the same pace no matter how hard we try, because that becomes unfair to James also. There's a fine balance between giving him all the opportunities and experiences that other children get, and making sure that we keep his routine enough for him to get optimal nutrition and sleep to continue to thrive. And having a few "off" days doesn't simply mean that we go back to normal and James goes back to normal. It can take days to weeks for him to find that normal again and balance out.

I'm pretty results driven. I don't mind hard work when I can see the results. I think that's why occasionally I crash. The constant work doesn't end, ever. He relies on me for literally everything. I feed him, bathe him, dress him, groom him, all his mobility is dependent upon me. So when I put so much effort into something, and see it failing, again and again, I fall apart a little bit. I have been struggling with James' weight and food for years, with no practical help.

It's hard to be honest as a caregiver without people thinking that you are whining. That is why you either always hear it from some people, because they are screaming out for a little bit of understanding and safety, that they are obviously not finding, or, you never hear it. I fall into that category. I don't want to be seen as weak, or failing, or needy, or whiney. But having a child with such high needs is exhausting. It won't go away. It won't get better. It's going to get harder and harder every year. There's no end in sight. And no answers as to how you are going to make the future work.

Once you voice that there is no end in sight, you deal with the guilt of having even thought that. Raising James is such a privilege and I am so thankful that he was entrusted to me. I am so thankful for the joy that he is. I don't ever want it to end; the thought of losing him is unfathomable.

But I need to fall sometimes. And feeling like I'm failing is a part of that. The struggle is constant and grueling with little peace. The feeling of failure has another side though. It reminds me of how much I love him. It reminds me that I love him to a depth that I never would have known had I not been given him. It reminds me that he has given me the strength of compassion, which keeps me going when life is hard and disgusting.

Every new mom imagines that perfect life. A cute house, white picket fence, a husband that works 9-5, fun family holidays, peaceful bedtimes and quiet nights, frilly aprons and conversation filled family meals, small children filling your house with laughter, play dates, birthday parties, perfectly dyed hair and painted nails, time to hit a gym, and hours spent with friends each week. I deal with puke, poop, boogies, and lack of sleep every day, all day. It's not a stage, it won't change, and it is getting significantly harder. The compassion keeps me going when projectile vomit has filled his eyes, nose, hit the carpet, and couch, my face, hands and clothes. The compassions keeps me going when we go to church, or out for a meal, and he decides to have a bowel movement. That is an immediate deal breaker. He is so unpleasant to be near when this is happening. He pushes up, stiffens up, makes the loudest, grossest poop pushing noises you can imagine. And then there's the smell. He isn't a baby anymore. It is rank. Like keel over, make you wanna throw up rank. We go home, or at least back to the van, when he poops. The compassion keeps me going when I have to clear the boogies out of his nose. If friends or family are over I also hear about how disgusting I am for doing this. Usually I am fine with that. But sometimes I'm seconds from losing my shit on them. I'm pretty sure when I wake up in the morning I don't say to myself, "yes, I get to pick someone else's nose today". And you are now thinking, oh my goodness, you pick his nose? With your finger? And you might be rethinking inviting me to dinner ☺

    Yes, I do. Why not use a Kleenex? Because it doesn't work. The boogies don't come out. He breathes through his nose while he chews on his hands, so his nose is so dry all of the time. They are dried and stuck in there. Why not use a saline? We have some, but he then breathes it right in, swallows it, and pukes because it's salt! Why not use a spray that is gentler than saline? We have that too. He still panics, breathes it in, and chokes and cries. Why not use a boogie sucker? We have one, and they are a joke! They really only work if you are dealing with snot and goopy gaggy type boogers. And no, gaggy is not a word, but when you deal with disgusting things all day, you are entitled to make up your own versions of words to describe your experiences.

So sometimes I feel like a failure because of the nagging comments that I hear, usually from people who love me and mean nothing by it. And usually I take nothing from it. My skin has gotten pretty thick over the years. But it builds up, and sometimes I need encouragement. A random kind word. To hear that even though everything is gross, disgusting, unpleasant, unwelcoming, and exhausting, what I am doing has value, and I am doing it well. Because I forget that when I'm in the routine of it all. I forget that I am giving him a dignity that many do not receive. I forget that I am doing it well.

The Lighter Side

The other side to being a parent who is a full time caregiver, is life when that child is not with you. I'm not talking about leaving the house for an hour or two without children. I am talking about several days without that child that is fully dependent on you.

Sometimes that looks like dropping them off at respite for a week, a service which we used to have access to. Because of where we are now living, we no longer have access to this. Or it may look like leaving both children with your spouse and going away for a weekend or longer with a girl friend. Or it may look like your dependent child going off to a special needs camp for a week, leaving you a week to spend with your "normal" child while your spouse works.

In all of those scenarios, there is a freedom that you cannot fully explain to someone who is not a caregiver. There is not anyone needing you for survival. And there won't be the next day. Or maybe even the next day. Now yes, all children need their parents for survival. But not in the way that James needs me.

There is an instant lightening of my heart, followed by a guilt. A guilt for how free I am feeling. How unburdened I am feeling for the days where he is not with me. I am noticing how easy life is when no one is depending on me for their quality of life. And not even for their quality of life; really, James depends on me for life.

I forget how easy it is to go out, when your child can get themselves ready, walk themselves out to the van, get in themselves, talk, and eat normal foods by themselves. It is like a vacation. How awful to say that not having James for a few days is like a vacation hey? Who says that about their child? Well, if all parents were honest, I think we all feel that way about our children from time to time. Or maybe several times a day, depending on the stage they are in! But man, if you are also a caregiver, you know exactly what I am talking about.

There is a stress that is always present when you are a caregiver. Your time is not your own. Your heart is not your own. Your mind is not your own. Your body is not your own. My body aches from lifting his 47 pound body up from the floor several times a day. Carrying him in and out of the van. Lifting his slippery body in and out of the tub. My mind belongs to his needs. I am always thinking about what he will eat at the next meal and the prep never ends. If he got enough calories. I am thinking about what he might be thinking or feeling but cannot express. I am constantly doing his laundry. My heart is burdened with realities that other people cannot see.

The other side to the daily grind of being a caregiver, is when I'm not a caregiver. And I feel free. But slightly lost in it all. It is overwhelming how easy life can become when he is not home, or I leave for a vacation. It is unnerving how light my heart can feel in an instant knowing that I have a break from caring for him. To be just me, only me, all me. To be able to sleep without knowing that I am always on call if he starts to choke, or his body violently jerks and scares him wide awake.

It takes a day or two to fully remember who I am without him, and then it seems that my time away is coming to a close! And I almost dread giving it up. I dread giving up the ability yo sleep soundly and without worry. I dread going back to the lifting. I dread the stress of his nutrition.

And yet, I wouldn't be me if I walked away from all of this to keep my freedom. I love nourishing his body with pureed food, lifting his body around with me to give him a high quality of life, taking care of all his hygiene needs so that others can see the handsome little charmer that he is.

Who he is, and all his needs, somehow completes who I am supposed to be. But man, that freedom. And yet, I dread the day when that freedom is every day. And the loneliness and grief that will carry. And I know that I will yearn to sacrifice that freedom forever, to have him back. Which brings back the guilt of feeling that freedom for short periods.

But if I were honest, that freedom rejuvenates me and keeps me going. I take breaks a few times a year with no children. And I am not nieve, I know that people think I am very selfish for doing this. But at home, and I on duty twenty four -seven, to an extent that will never be understood by someone who has not stepped into a caregivers role for an extended period. And I cherish these times. So yes, the freedom may be viewed as selfish; but if you knew the reality of never ending care, you would understand the meaning of that freedom.

We have recently lost our access to respite. Before moving, we qualified for six weeks of respite a year, for free, at Wascana Rehabilitation in Regina, Saskatchewan. We never used that much, but it was such a blessing to have this service available to us. They had a pediatric respite ward, with five beds, and two or three staff at all times. The criteria to receive this respite was that your child was tube fed and lived in southern Saskatchewan.

James is not ever a burden to me, but I did not realize the weight I was carrying until he was away in respite. I did not realize the constant pressure and responsibility I was under until that was not there. To sleep through the night without a monitor buzzing in my ear all night was bliss! To wake up in the morning and not have to change his diaper, his clothes, wash him up, brush his teeth, tube feed him, and orally feed him, all before getting myself ready, felt so odd. To have a free evening once Julia was in bed, and not have to stay up trying to get James to sleep was almost awkward at first. I had no idea what to do!

I would use respite services when I would travel to Calgary for oncology appointments, or when we were going away for a few days, and Julia would go to her grandparents or stay with a friend.

Having some form of respite in place is critical to doing this long term. Whether that's somewhere that formally offers respite services, a family member, or someone you pay to come into your home for a few days at a time. If you cannot find the services to allow for overnight care, even scheduling very regular time away in few hour long segments lets you know a short break is always near and you can make it through. Time away refreshes and energizes.

Our first respite experiences were a complete disaster! It took so long for things to go well and for me to relax enough to enjoy the reprieve. But it is so worth sticking with it, and finding a respite option that works for you, your child, and your family.

{2011}

James started school full time in September 2011, two months shy of turning four years old. We lived 15 minutes out of town from his school, and I drove him into school and picked him up each day. He finally began to love school! Now instead of crying when I left, he would cry when I picked him up. Which made the end of every day rather miserable, as he would often cry the entire way home also. But dropping him off at school had become so easy. Although it would have been nice if he at least took the time to wave as I left! He was so engrossed with what his friends were doing the second that we got into the school that it was like I simply disappeared. A good problem to have after the previous year of school hell!

He really started to make social progress this year. Instead of being tied to mommy all day every day, he was learning to trust his teachers and aides, although we still needed to be careful with change. The general structure of the program was that each child would work with many different aides throughout the day. James was having a lot of trouble adapting to so much change; he really requires predictable structure. So his days became a lot more structured, with a consistent few educational assistants working with him each day.

James gained confidence in being away from me this year, and slowly learned how to have relationships with other adults that he came to trust. Routine was still key, but we were making huge strides.

This year was filled with highs and lows, and never ending hard work. We went on James' wish trip to DisneyWorld, and I was diagnosed with cancer.

Wish trip

In January of 2011 we started the process with the Make-A-Wish Foundation of Saskatchewan. Along with the excitement that comes with this, comes a harsh reality. We were only able to apply for this wish because our child had a life shortening illness. I worried that they wouldn't see his congenital cytomegalovirus and cerebral palsy as life shortening, and the last thing I wanted to do was to argue for a gift. If we were turned down that was it – we would not appeal it.

We filled out the paperwork, and sent it in. It took a few weeks, as they contacted his neonatologist, as cCMV is not something many doctors are highly educated in. Then the call came, "we are so sorry for how long the process took, but we would be honored to grant a wish for James." I remember that phone call like it was yesterday. She was so kind, and soft spoken, but so excited! I cried tears of joy, and once we hung up, the tears fast turned to tears of grief. We got approved awfully easily, because James' life is expected to be too short.

None the less, we started to dream. Do we do something now, or wait until he is older and can understand it more and remember it? Should we go somewhere? Or get something that he could use every day at home? We tossed around the idea of a hot tub, or indoor therapy pool; basically an indoor hot tub. James' muscles loosen so much in hot water, and we would use that for him every day! We would all benefit from that every day. And we talked about a trip. A trip would go so fast, but it would be for everyone. A much needed break from the day to day reality we lived in. A break to reconnect as a family, and just laugh. However, he was only three years old, he wouldn't remember it. And Julia was only 5 years old, so her memories would also be vague.

How do you decide on something like this? James cannot understand what we are trying to decide, and he cannot communicate to us what his wish would be. So how do we make the very best decision for him? We asked ourselves a few questions. If we wait, will we wait too long? James was healthy and strong right now, something we know can be taken away very quickly without any warning. Is it better to gamble with waiting, or to live in the right now, and take full advantage of the current healthy state that he was in? We chose to live in the present and start planning our wish for James!

We met with our wish coordinator in Saskatoon, and after some long discussion, we chose to plan a trip to DisneyWorld! Blue cross waives the pre-existing medical condition clause for wish kids, so this was the only trip we would ever be able to take out of Canada with full medical coverage. This made the decision quite easy. We looked at what James' favorite things include: his sister, watching people, being in the sun, and swimming.

We had the choice to stay on resort at Disney, or at Give Kids the World. Immediately, we thought, Disney of course! But after some advice from others who had been on a wish trip, we chose Give Kids the World. GKTW is a resort in Kissimmee Florida, dedicated solely to sick kids coming to Florida on a wish trip. They provide you with a half duplex to live in for the week, all meals, rides, swimming, spray park, train ride, theatre, parades, all day ice cream, constant street parties, fully wheelchair accessible outdoor playground themed as candyland, and so much more! Disney characters come out every day from Disney, and they have many of their own princess' and characters.

Blog Entry {February 26, 2011} Make a Wish!

  The second week of January we received a call from The Children's Wish Foundation. They were giving James a wish! Quite honestly, a very bitterly sweet moment for us as parents. We were overwhelmed that through others generosity, our child was going to receive a gift that we would likely never be able to give! And at the same time, it meant that James met the criteria for a wish..... a lift shortening illness. And unlike many other things, there is no cure.
  We went to Saskatoon this last week, and James made a wish! Well, we made a wish for him! How do you make a wish for a little boy who has no way to tell us what he would want to do? We took into consideration his very favorite things in life.... his sister, his family, being outside, watching children, and swimming. We took into consideration that this was a family memory that we will always cherish. And what was the decision - DISNEYWORLD!
  The kids had a blast playing with Roary the Wish Lion while we were there! We got a smaller version of Roary to take home, and they are taking turns sleeping with him each night. We have the privilege of staying at a resort called Give Kids the World. It is for wish kids from around the world.

  Our coordinator planned all the details, and booked our trip for May of 2011. We flew from Saskatoon to Colorado, where we had a two hour layover to get through customs and get back through security and onto our next flight. Which is LOTS of time! Unless you have a tube fed, non verbal, wheelchair bound child. We got held up in security for an hour, while they swabbed all his enteral food, oral food, and medications, his g-tube, and his wheelchair. I pleaded with them to please hurry, showing them which gate we needed to get to, and our flight time, to which they replied, "You will make your flight ma'am". We ran through the airport, caught the underground train, ran through the airport some more, ran on the moving sidewalks, and got to our gate just as they locked the large steel door. And in a shining moment of strength, I crumpled like a small child on the floor and cried. Embarassing in hind sight! But so needed in that moment!! United got us on a flight two hours later, the kids waited well, and we still made it to Orlando that day.

    A volunteer from Give Kids the World met us at the airport, even though we were arriving two hours later than expected, took us to our rental van, and gave us directions to the resort. We were greeted there with a stuffed Mickey Mouse for James, a stuffed Shamu for Julia, and the keys to our home for the next 7 nights. It was right across from candyland park, and absolutely charming! It had a nice kitchen, a large living room, and two bedrooms. Our bedroom had a king size bed and a tv. The kids' room had two single beds, and a huge ensuite bathroom, all wheelchair accessible with a roll in shower and a large jetted tub. They had bedrails for James' bed there for us, a highchair for feeding, and all the diapers, wipes, and formula we would need while we were there. We also had our own washer and dryer, which is incredible when you have a drooling, puking, diapered child.

    The next day they give you an orientation, where you get all of the information needed for things going on at Give Kids the World, your Disney park hopper passes, Universal studio passes, sea world passes, and you can choose from a whole book of other places to go for free. Knowing James would tire easily and swimming was so much fun for him, we didn't plan a lot. We used our three days at Disney, and did one day at Sea World. We shopped downtown Disney one day, and spent the remainder of our time at Give Kids the World. With the exception of the evenings we stayed late at Magic Kingdom and Epcot for the fireworks, we were back at GKTW everyday for supper and to spend our evening swimming in their amazing water park.

Our Disney days were spent at Magic Kingdom, Animal Kingdom, Epcot, and Hollywood Studios. We did a full day at Magic Kingdom, with our favorite attractions being: Pirates of the Caribbean, Splash Mountain, Big Thunder Railroad rollercoaster, it's a small world, Peter Pan's flying adventure and Space mountain. James' favorites were it's a small world and Peter Pan, both being slower rides with so much to look at. Any ride that we loaded him onto we had the option of staying on for two rounds, which was really nice considering how long it took to safely get him on and off in most cases. We stayed late at Magic Kingdom to get ice cream and watch the fireworks, which everyone really enjoyed.

We only spent half a day at Animal Kingdom, with the highlights being: Expedition Everest, Finding Nemo – the musical, Kali River Rapids, and Kilimanjaro Safari. We found Animal Kingdom to be small and so over crowded, making it hard to maneuver with James without becoming very frustrated.

We only spent half a day at Epcot, and we could have spent a whole day there very easily. The top attractions were: Soarin and Test Track. We spent a lot of our time walking through the pavilions, then got some supper and found a nice place to sit and watch IllumiNations, the fireworks and water show. The pavilions are authentic and breathtaking. You feel as if you have stepped inside the country for a few short minutes. Everything is intricately planned and executed. The buildings tower over you; they are majestic and delightful. I felt like a small child, in awe with each new country that we walked through. After the fireworks show you can walk around the lake, after all the pavilions have closed for the day, and simply take in their beauty. Don't try this in Magic Kingdom though as they will chase you out!! (not that we had this experience;)

Our day spent at Hollywood Studios was loved by everyone. Our highlights included: Beauty and the Beast show, Indiana Jones stunt show, The Great Movie Ride, and Tower of Terror. Toy Story Mania was a favorite for all of us; we rode it so many times and every time everyone was laughing throughout the ride. If you are on a wish trip, simply mention that when you enter through the exit of the shows; sometimes they will ask if you would like a meet and greet with the cast afterwards, and if they don't, just simply ask if it is possible. We did this with both Finding Nemo and the Indiana Jones Stunt show, which was really neat for all of us.

We spent a day at Sea World also. Disney treated us very well with our Wish Child buttons, but Sea World went above and beyond. The only ride we did there was Atlantis, but we entered through the exit, and they immediately loaded us. For the Shamu show, they took us in before they started admitting the public, and we could pick where we would like to be seated. James got to feed the dolphins, and again, they took him in the exit before admitting anyone else, and a trainer gave us the fish and allowed us all the time we needed to put it into his hands and let him feed the dolphins. He was mesmerized on the moving sidewalks in the tunnels through the aquariums with the fish and sharks swimming all around us.

Downtown Disney is beautifully set on water, with all kinds of shops and restaurants to visit. We did a little bit of shopping, took some pictures, and had a fun lunch at the Rainforest Cafe. Julia was a little unsure of the thunderstorm while we were eating but enjoyed the monkeys! James spent his time taking it all in, and laughing at the animal noises.

However, by far, the highlight of this trip for everyone, was Give Kids the World. Not only did they go out of their way to treat James just like every other child, they also made a point to make Julia feel like she was just as special on this trip. The meals were healthy and delicious, with so many options that the kids liked also. The cooks were always very accommodating with James, and came out to offer him yogurts and puddings from the back at the lunch and supper meals when they weren't on the buffets. Both Julia and James got tattoos done in the spa, and Julia had her nails done. They both also loved to ride the carousel almost every time we walked by it! They had pirate and princess parties, parades, Christmas once a week complete with Santa and snow and presents. Every day they came in to clean our villa, and a gift would be left on the table for each of the kids. We had the option to order from Boston Market once a day, and we could pick it up in the "downtown square", or call and have it delivered to our villa. The ice cream parlour was open early each morning until late each evening; on our last day there we even indulged in ice cream for breakfast. Mayor Clayton and Miss Merry were the GKTW mascots, and they came to tuck our kids into bed one night, which was a highlight for Julia, but I think James was a little concerned at the large animal that was trying to tuck him in for the night!

James' sleep habits, throwing up, crying, and tightness were all concerns for us on this trip. Would it all be far too overwhelming for him? Would anyone manage to get any sleep? As it turned out, the hot humid air, mixed with constant family time, was the perfect recipe for him. His muscles relaxed, he did not throw up, and he slept all night every night. He was usually asleep before he even got his medicine. He ate well at meal times, and we gave him fluids via g-tube throughout the day when we were out in the sun to keep him hydrated. He laughed all day everyday at all the kids everywhere, and he just loved every second of being with his family.

We spent all but two of our evenings at GKTW. We would have supper, go for a nice walk, and then hit the pool until bedtime. James would laugh like crazy while we swam, mostly at his sister. Julia had so much fun, and James just loved watching her swim. I think everyone in the village knew when we came out of the pool each night, by his blood curdling screams! He hated when it was time to get out, he would cry all the way back to our villa, which was a five minute walk. And within minutes of getting inside, that screaming boy was sound asleep for the night.
It was heaven to see him so happy all day. To see his muscles loose and not fighting him. To see Julia just being a kid, and not having her day planned around what James' needs are at home. To all be together all day, having fun, and then see them sleep so soundly. To have the stress of the medical needs taken off us as parents for a week, and have those sweet children catered to and spoiled; a once in a lifetime trip, that we never wanted to need, but are so grateful to have had the opportunity.

Looking back, we sometimes think, should we have waited? James is seven now, and doing the best physically that he has ever done. And his comprehension of what is going on around him is so high. But no, we should not have waited. We had no way of knowing he would be so strong four years later. We are deeply thankful for the week we had, away from the weight of caring for his needs, making memories that we treasure to this day.

If you can take anything from our experience, please don't forget, that families who are receiving these wishes, while their thankfulness is overflowing, their hearts are hurting for why it is needed. Lend a sincere hug.

If you are a family with a highly dependent child, heading out on a big trip, or even a wish trip, here are a few tips to make travelling a little bit easier.

- If you are going on a wish trip, arrange to have all supplies such as: special feeding formulas, diapers, wipes at your destination when you get there. That saves a whole suitcase.
- We did not bring our big metal wheelchair. Instead we brought his special tomato pushchair. We did not label his chair clearly as a wheelchair, but if we ever fly with him again it will be labelled as such. Having large labels will just save the constant explaining that your child cannot walk and this isn't merely a stroller. Disney will place their own label on it for this purpose.
- Pre board your plane as soon as the call is made. As you are getting settled, speak with one of your flight attendants. Explain your child's situation and needs to them, and ask if they can make accommodations during your flight for you to lie them somewhere to change them. They are usually quite willing to accommodate you – but if you are making the request once the plane is full and they are in the full swing of their routine, it will be harder to accommodate. You will also end up explaining all of the details in front of everyone sitting around you, which can be avoided by having the conversation earlier.
- Don't over plan your days. The constant over stimulation can become overwhelming. We planned two evenings away from our resort, and the rest of the week we stayed on resort for the evenings. He

always got enough sleep and our days were very successful.
- We chose not to bring our feeding pump. We knew that our days would be very busy, so we simply kept his extension attached to his mic-key button, and kept water and formula in an insulted bag attached to the wheelchair and every hour I gave him a few syringes of both formula and water. Kept him perfectly hydrated in the heat, never hungry, and less equipment to haul around with us. It also meant we changed diapers all day long ☺
- Any parks/places you go for the day, scope out places to feed and change immediately. Ask at the gate, or go to an administration or first aid building. If your child no longer fits on a baby changing table, if you explain your situation, you can often make arrangements to use an office or a first aid room as you need throughout the day. Whether it's a clean floor or a first aid cot, as long as it comes with some privacy, it is so much better than trying to change them in a public washroom.
- Carry as little food with you as possible in your carry on, and give yourself plenty of time to get through security. We missed a flight because they had to swab all of his formula, his wheelchair, and even his actual mic-key button. Because he was unable to speak and answer any of their questions about someone possibly hiding something on him or his chair, their search of him had to be very thorough.
- Carry any doctor's notes that pertain to your child's care in their passport. We had a note in ours stating that because of his medical condition, it was impossible to get his picture to the passport standards and this was good enough. Also, that he requires the mic-key button for feeding, and that he

took medication and formula through it, which we would be carrying with us in our carry on.
- Take your pharmacies contact information with you just in case a prescription medication is lost somehow. This way they can fax it to a pharmacy where you are and save you a doctor visit.
- If your child has a feeding tube, bring an extra. I brought an extra tube, and a catheter just in case the backup button failed.
- Do over pack on medical supplies – that way you are prepared for anything that could go wrong. Don't over pack on everyday things that you can just buy – clothes, diapers...

Cancer

"It's just a rare cancer, we will need to do another surgery." And he then turned and left the room.

Before we left for our wish trip, I had a minor procedure done to remove a cyst from the back of my skull. My family doctor has assured me it was merely a cyst a year before, but it hurt, and was growing, and I asked to have it removed. It was a bump under my skin, which did move slightly when touched, but still seemed to be attached to the skull. He tried to do it in our local hospital, but once he opened it up he realized a plastic surgeon should be doing it. Also, the freezing he gave me didn't take, so I felt him cut my scalp open! Thank God I brought a friend with me who knew instantly that something was not ok! I completely went to another place mentally to cope and I think she did all the talking – I actually don't remember clearly! So I waited eight months to get in to see a plastic surgeon, and have it removed.

Two large needles were stuck into my head to freeze the area. If you have ever had a needle in your head you will know exactly the shudder that goes through me when I say that. Not only can you feel the needles enter, and feel the medicine being pushed into your head, you can also hear it, from the inside. It's a nails on a chalk board times a million kind of feeling!

Once the freezing had taken, about 20 minutes later, he returned, and made about an inch long cut in my scalp. Again, I could hear this, on the inside. It sounded like styrofoam being cut while yours ears were popping and filling with water at the same time. It was absolutely sick! He tried to simply pop it out like it should have, but it would not budge. It took him quite a while of scraping and cutting to get it, all the while blood was dripping down my neck onto the bed beside me, creating quite a large pool and soaking through several towels. Slightly unnerving! After quite a while he said they got it all and sewed me back up.

I asked to see what they took from me, so he brought me a plastic cup that they had put it into. Gross! It was grey, with faded spots, and looked like a brain! It was about the size of a whopper candy. He said it would be sent to pathology just to be sure, but everything should be good! My stitches would dissolve themselves and I wouldn't need any more follow up. Perfect!

So off we went on our wish trip the next month! When we returned home, my plastic surgeons number was on my phone, so I called them back, and the receptionist asked me to come back for some results. Some results? They don't call for good news. Still, we didn't really think it could be much. Up until now I had to fight for what care I did get.

My husband came with me, and we went to Regina, both pretty nervous. The receptionist called us into a room, and we waited. Finally my surgeon's intern entered the room. He casually looks at me, and says, "It's just a rare cancer, we will need to do another surgery." And he then turned and left the room, closing the door behind him.

What?? We both looked at each other and were like, he didn't just say that I have cancer and then walk out did he?! What the hell!! So we waited. Pretty quietly. Then we heard my surgeon "quietly yelling" at him! "You never go into a room, tell someone they have cancer, and then walk out!!" He sounded pretty angry!

So, enter my surgeon, after what felt like an eternity. First, he apologized for what just happened. Then he continued to say that yes, the cyst was a cancer. It was called DFSP, dermatofibrosarcoma protuberance. A very very rare cancer, about one in a million cancers will be this one. He described that this tumor grows tentacles, and it would be spreading out away from what they removed, and I would require a wide excision. They would remove a larger area of tissue, everything right down to my skull, in about a three inch diameter circle, and do a skin graft from my left thigh to close it back up. The hospital would call me to arrange the surgery.

We left the office, and I stood in an alley downtown Regina, and called my best friend Christine. She answered, and I responded with, "Hey, wanna go wig shopping with me?" Let me just say, if you ever find yourself in a similar situation, humor is not always the answer! She was so very mad at me. I told her all that I knew, and we both cried. We went home, and that evening I drove into Saskatoon to tell my parents and sister. Christine came to my parents and spent the night with me, and I drove home the next day. And now I had to tell Julia.

I couldn't really tell James. I could, but he would probably just laugh and hit me!! But Julia, how do we do this honestly and without fear? Well, we decided that the best way to take the fear out of it was to tell her immediately, and to be completely honest. It's amazing how much they really can take in. We sat down with her, told her that the cyst was actually cancer, told her about the surgery, and asked if she had any questions. She asked if I would be ok, and we told her that the doctors were very sure that they should be able to remove it all with the surgery. And with that she went off to play! Haha!

Later that week I went to Julia's school to meet with her teacher. We lived in a small community, and I knew some of her friends would have heard, and I wanted to make sure her teacher knew. Cancer can be a scary word for children, often associated with the death of grandparents, and I was worried that it would be talked about, without the presence of an adult, and she would become scared. He watched in the classroom, and made sure any talk was done openly and without fear of death.

The hospital called the day after my appointment with a surgery date, just a week and a half after my appointment. She apologized for how far away the surgery was and how long I was having to wait, and was so kind. I thought that was incredibly fast to be going in for surgery!

Fast forward to the night before my surgery. Since they were going to be removing so much tissue from my head and doing a graft, and I wouldn't be able to get my head wet for weeks, I opted to simply shave my head. It would make things so much neater and less risk of infection. So, in my bathroom, me, John, and Christine, all stood around the clippers. First I was quite giggly, from nerves. Then, as I turned on that razor, it hit me. I started out doing it, and the tears started shortly after, feeling my hair hit the floor. It all felt so surreal. Not because I was shaving my head, but because I had cancer. John left a few minutes in, it was too real. I handed the razor to Christine after about half my head was done. We were both crying, but she kissed my forehead, and finished what I had started but couldn't finish . My mom and sister were coming from Saskatoon to stay with the kids for my surgery, so I wanted it done before they arrived.

The morning of, John, Christine and I were out the door before the kids were up for the day, leaving them with my mom and sister. I was lying on a stretcher in day surgery in the Pasqua hospital in Regina, waiting to be wheeled into surgery. They didn't give me any relaxants before I went in, however, no one else would have known that! I was absolutely ridiculous! I was more entertaining than someone who was grossly intoxicated! All from nerves! I was soooooo cold, so they brought me this huge inflatable blanket, that was constantly filling with hot air. Well, I was lying with this thing on me, holding my hands just below my chest, exclaiming to the world that I now had eight enormous boobies! Over and over again. Thank goodness I didn't know anybody there!

Finally they came to get me, wheeled me into a white very cold room, got me to lie on my back on the narrowest table ever, and put a mask over my face. And obviously that is all I remember! I still have an unanswered question though; how did they get me onto my stomach to do the surgery without dropping me on the floor?! I've never asked, because I'm assuming I don't want to know the answer.

I remember partially waking up to people in my face, trying to get me to talk. I couldn't keep my eyes open long enough to really see them, never mind talk to them. I saw Christine's face and went back to sleep. John had went for a walk. Then I remember a nurse telling me I had to walk to the bathroom before I could go home. I tried to tell her I couldn't, but she grabbed me, pulled me up, hauled me to the bathroom, then was annoyed that she needed to help me up and get me back to bed after! She discharged me right then. I couldn't keep my eyes open, communicate, or walk on my own, but they needed my bed. My helpers wheeled me to the van in a wheelchair, somehow got me in the back, and I just remember falling asleep on Christine on the back bench, and then I was home. There is no way I should have been discharged so soon, I definitely couldn't even stand on my own yet.

My mom and sister stayed the next day to make sure everything around the house was caught up. Christine mostly stayed with me, we watched The Sweetest Thing in bed! John balanced working and almost everything with the kids. My recovery itself went very well. I stayed on top of my pain meds so nothing ever got too severe. The antibiotics unfortunately made me so sick. I was on something very strong to ensure no infection set in, but my stomach could not handle them. I'm not really sure why I took them because I'm sure I threw almost every single dose back up. Once those were done in two weeks I began to feel much better!

Life pretty much returned to normal. Three days after my surgery we could pull off the gauze. I had a 3 inch wide crater on the back of my head, surrounded by 52 staples. And a 3 inch by 5 inch donor skin site on my thigh, which was covered in gauze, plastic, and lots of tape. Maybe I should have shaved there properly first?! Oops!

Two weeks after my surgery, while I was getting my first batch of staples removed from the head, my surgeon informed me that all was good and no further treatment was needed. I remember the breath I took after he said those words! I was so relieved! I think I told everyone I knew my good news within minutes of hearing it. Life could go on without the fear of cancer. I wore scarves on my head to cover my baldness and my surgery site until it was healed. Once it was healed I purchased a wig to wear until more of my hair came back.

For no reason at all, in September, I suddenly didn't feel quite right about how my pathology results had been shared with me. My surgeon never came into the room and exclaimed the good news! Rather, I found him in the hallway and asked, and he said "oh ya, you're all good, no more treatment is needed." I'm not sure why, but all of a sudden this struck me as odd. That day I called his office and asked for a hard copy of those pathology results, and I drove in the next day to get them.

If you've ever seen a pathology report, you know there's a lot of information on there that is hard to understand when you are looking at it for the first time. However, one thing stuck out to me, "deep margin remains positive." From here I went to my DFSP support group online, to find out if that meant what I thought it meant; that they didn't get all the cancer. I still had cancer. I still had cancer?? They confirmed my fears; I still had cancer. I was enraged! My hands were shaking, my voice was raspy. My head was foggy. My balance was gone.

The first thing I did was call the cancer clinic. Surely I should have an oncologist at this point right? I asked my surgeon before my surgery if I should be seeing one, and he said that wasn't necessary, he could take care of everything himself. Well, the cancer clinic informed me that I absolutely should be seeing an oncologist, however, they were unable to see me without a referral from the diagnosing doctor. This nurse also informed me that by law, my surgeon was required to refer me over to them as soon as a diagnosis of cancer was made with that initial pathology report.

This is probably a good time to sit down and think things through before venting all your anger right? So naturally, I immediately dialed up my surgeon's office and probably said some things I would take back today, if only I could actually remember them. What I do remember from that conversation is the receptionist. She was incredibly gracious. She already knew what was coming when I told her who I was. I suddenly remembered that when I came in for that report, she went to the back, and I could hear her talking angrily. I was putting the pieces together, she definitely knew that he should have contacted me. That something slipped through that shouldn't have. Bless this lady.

She made me an appointment to return later that week to see him. When he walked into the office, my mind was reeling. But I bit my tongue, controlled my attitude, and gave him the benefit of the doubt. I asked why he told me that I needed no further treatment, why the report stated that my deep margin remained positive, and why no referral to the cancer clinic was ever made on my behalf. He immediately got defensive, and even began to raise his voice. He actually refused to give me a referral, stating that "it was only a little bit of cancer left." Things turned a little less than pretty at this point. Excuse me?? What the hell did you just say to me?? Lucky for me, I was far enough in my journey with James to know how to get what I need, and the fight was on. I walked out of that office having the written referral, and having watched the receptionist call over to the cancer clinic in front of me, explain the situation, and fax off the referral in front of my very eyes.

I left exhausted. Why did I just need to fight to see an oncologist when I still had cancer? And angry. I was so angry. Why was I lied to? Why would you tell someone that they were cancer free, when they were not?

I got a call from Lynn, my nurse at the cancer clinic, the next day, and an appointment was made within the next week. So I drove back into Regina by myself for another appointment. There's something completely unnerving about walking into a cancer clinic for the first time ever, by yourself, not having a clue what to expect from the day. Everything was white and sterile. The staff was overly cheery and bubbly. Annoyingly cheerful. And I was the youngest person, at 30 years old, by over 20 years easily. And that smell, you don't ever forget that sterile smell.

My name was called and I followed my nurse down the hallway, making pleasant small talk as we went. Stopping at the dreaded scale so she could record my weight. She took me to a small interior room, and had me sit down to wait for my oncologist. I was to see a radiation oncologist that day. The door opened, and in walked the nicest doctor. She looked me in the eye, shook my hand lovingly, and introduced herself. She then asked if I was alone today, and then went to get a social worker to sit with me. This got my heart racing. Why did I need someone to sit with me? Her name was Linda, and she was very sweet. My doctor started by explaining what it meant that my deep margin was still positive. They had removed all tissue right down to my skull, and a three inch circle, and it was against my skull where cancer cells were still found to be present. She then explained my options.

    I could have a surgery done where a large part of my skull would be removed, presenting many complications as they would be dealing with attached brain matter. Or, we could start radiation tomorrow. A high dose of radiation, five days per week, for six weeks. She then took my hand and explained that if we go with this option, I will die from brain cancer within 20 years. She sat silently for a moment, she could probably see the color draining from my face. She then moved her stool closer to me, and said that if I was her daughter, she would want me to go to Calgary, to the Tom Baker Cancer Clinic, where they have a sarcoma team, who could help me to make the best decision possible for me. She was not willing to give me that radiation unless they felt it was absolutely crucial; the best of two evils. There was no effective chemotherapy to fight this cancer.

    From there, Linda took me to pick out a new wig, hoping it would lighten my heart just for a moment. We picked out a beautiful dark longer straight hair wig, which I wore home from the clinic. I don't remember that hour long drive home. I made some phone calls before I left the hospital, but I don't remember them. I don't even remember the rest of the day. All I remember is the numbness. I still have cancer. And the radiation to cure it could kill me.

My appointment at the Tom Baker clinic in Calgary was four days later. We made all the arrangements for the kids, and went to Calgary. Somehow I felt peace with the situation as a whole. Walking into the Tom Baker felt surreal all over again. This place was huge!! All of these people have cancer? How can that be possible. So many people looked so scared. So many tears. So many empty stares. So many overly cheerful nurses.

The questionnaire before you see the doctor was two pages long. I felt like a cancer patient sitting filling out that form, among rows and rows of others, doing the very same thing. Eventually I was led to another waiting room, and after about an hour, to a small examination room. Doctors and nurses both came in and out, asking questions, touching my head, looking at the reports I had brought with me. Interns came in and repeated it all.

At the end, they explained that for the moment we were going to sit on it. Yes, there was still cancer according to my reports. First, they were going to order my actual slides from my surgery, and ensure that the original diagnosis was correct, that my deep margin was still positive, and that nothing else remained positive. They also ordered me a CT scan, to look for any more growth. Once the scan was done, and the slides had been reanalyzed by sarcoma specialists, my case would go before a sarcoma board, consisting of ten sarcoma specialists – radiation and surgical oncologists, pathologists, and nurses. From here, a treatment recommendation would be made.

We spent a night in Banff to offset the low mood of the appointment – a tradition that would be kept for sure! In Regina I had my CT done, and my results were given to me on a disc and I brought them with me back to Calgary, a few weeks later. This was the appointment where I would hear my options and they would make their recommendation. And their recommendation was this; do nothing. If we shoot radiation where it's needed, it also goes straight through to my brain, guaranteeing a brain cancer. It is also a one time deal; if I do the radiation now, we have no action plan if it returns. No chemo is available to treat this cancer. The surgery was too risky. I was needed at home for James – the risk was unnecessary. This cancer has a 50-80% reoccurrence rate, with or without the positive deep margin. Even with that radiation, I had a very high chance of this returning. They recommended that we simply watch. If it returned, it would most likely return to the same site, and because all tissue had been removed down to my skull, we would feel a tumor regrowing fairly fast. The chance of it spreading to other parts of the body are fairly low. If it does it will go to my lungs or lymph nodes. Very rarely will it penetrate bone, there have only been a few known cases where this has happened. I was too young to use our only fighting chance up now, and have nothing to battle with later if necessary. We felt a peace about that, and went with their recommendation.

  I am now three and half years past that surgery. I am thirty three years old now, with no signs of this returning yet. I am followed through the Regina cancer clinic once a year now, and the Tom Baker clinic once a year, with the option to call and book an appointment both places any time I think there's something we need to check out. I have had two more lumps on my head biopsied since my surgery, but both were negative.

  I would be lying if I said I always felt a peace about this. I can have peace about it, and still feel the reality about it. My body has been so different since this happened. I had viral encephalitis a year after my surgery, leaving me on my couch for four weeks, in and out of the hospital five times, at times completely unable to talk, to make eye contact, hardly able to move. It was like I was trapped in my body; I could see what was happening around me, but I was completely unable to respond to it. I was diagnosed with celiac disease shortly after this. My pain tolerance used to be incredibly high; now I seem to feel things differently. Deeper. Pain radiates through me like I have never experienced before. My anemia has gotten more severe. Simple sicknesses wipe me out. My hearing changed. Tests don't show any change, but I can no longer differentiate between foreground and background noise. My teeth have weakened. I have never had cavities before, and now I dread the dentist even more because no matter what I do, I always have cavities.

What has this journey done for me? It has made me take time, slow down, breathe in the small moments, find beauty in the simple things, and to let myself feel. It forces me to give my worry over to God, again, and again, and again. There are days where my nagging cough whispers at me that this could be the cancer spreading, and if so, it's likely too late for any effective treatment. Those lymph nodes in the back of my neck that like to swell up a few times a week since my surgery three and a half years ago, sometimes taunt me; what if it has spread. But I have to give that to my God, in complete confidence that He will work everything out. If my time comes sooner than I'd like it to, He will make provisions for my family.

This has taught me to treasure the moments that really matter. To put down the laundry that needs to be folded to snuggle with my daughter before bedtime. To walk away from the dishes to lie on the floor with James and hear his precious giggle.

I've further learnt to love people. To love them where they are at in their journey through whatever they may be walking through, whether I know what that trial is or not. Every person is struggling with something; no one has everything put together perfectly. Smile at people that you walk by. I try not to let my own insecurities about myself keep me from loving people genuinely.

I try to leave my heart open. This, together with having a very sensitive heart, can often lead to deep hurt. However, the hurt is ok, because that means that I am loving and feeling and living in the present. It is okay to hurt, as long as I don't stay there. As long as forgiveness overcomes that hurt, and love can still find its way through.

In 2014 I had a daffodil tattooed onto my left foot, in turquoise and purple, because I was scared a yellow foot tattoo would end up looking like a fungal disease in twenty years! This provided closure for me. I look down at the gorgeous tattoo everyday and it reminds me to be present in every moment.

Life is short. I want to be remembered for loving.

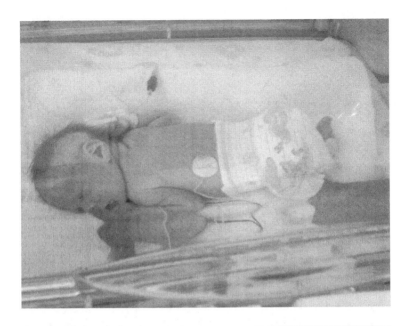

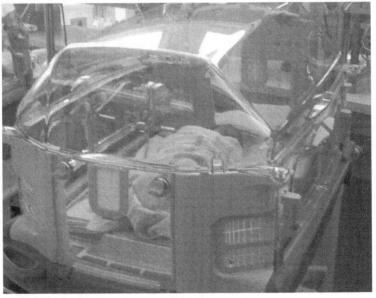

NICU

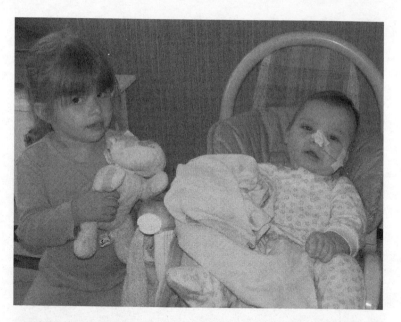

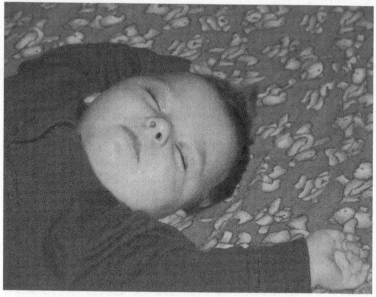

NG Tube / The first time James fell asleep alone, on the floor, September 2008

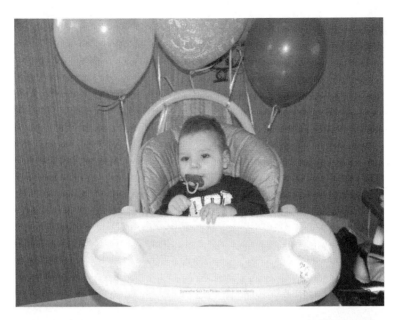

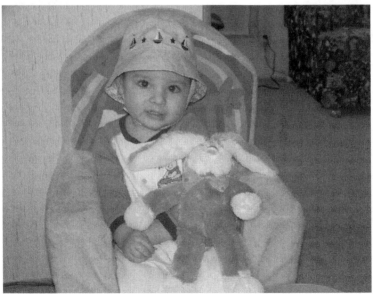

First Birthday / Easter 2009

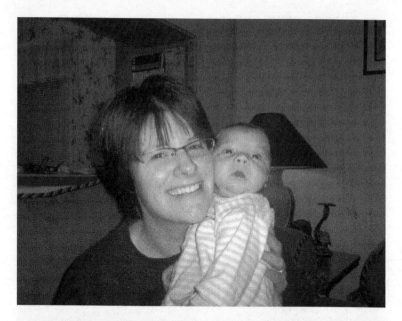

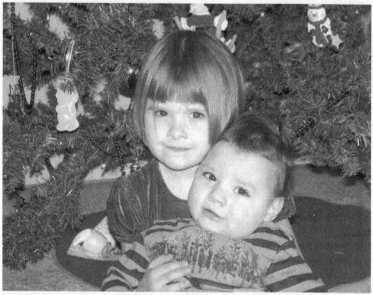

First Christmas / Second Christmas

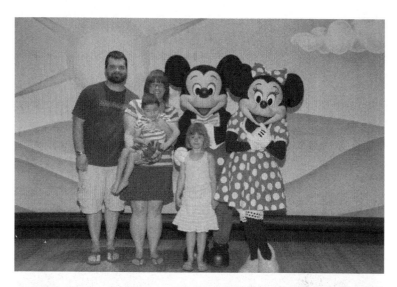

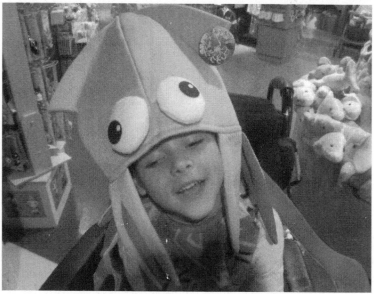

2011 – Wish Trip to DisneyWorld / 2013 – Trip to Mall of America – Nickelodeon

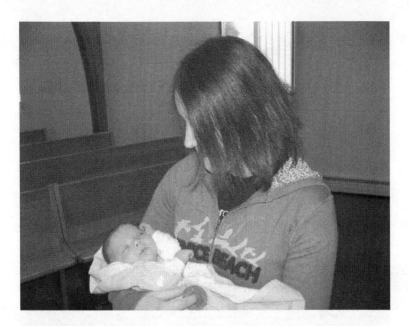

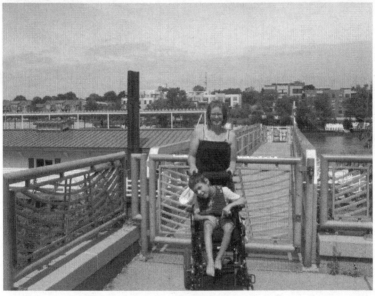

One month old / 2013 waiting to board a river boat on the Mississippi River

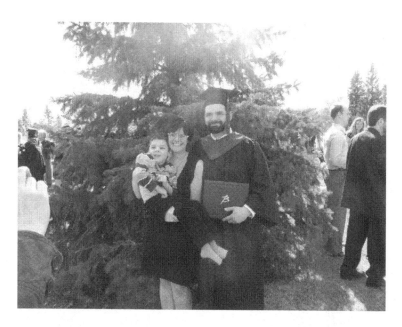

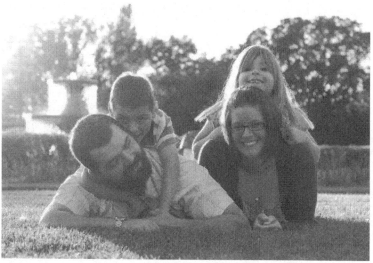

2012 – John's graduation from Briercrest / 2013 – Family Picture

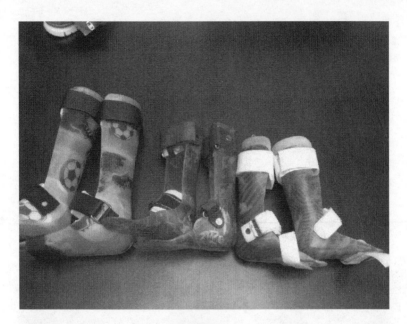

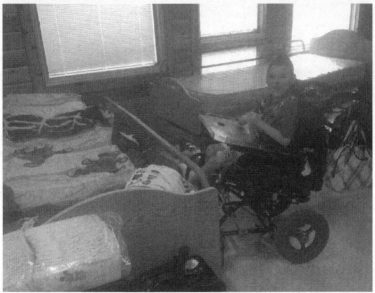

AFO's / First year at Camp Easter Seal 2014

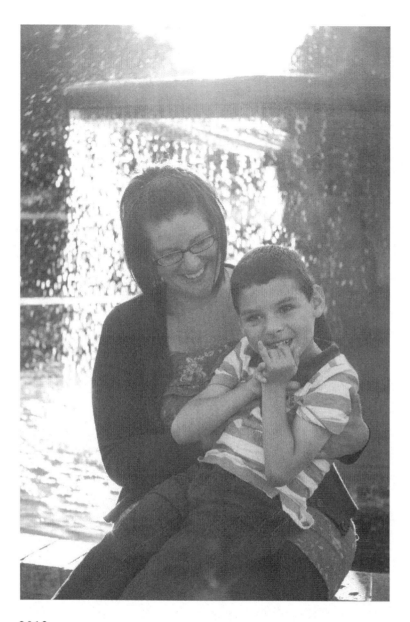

2013

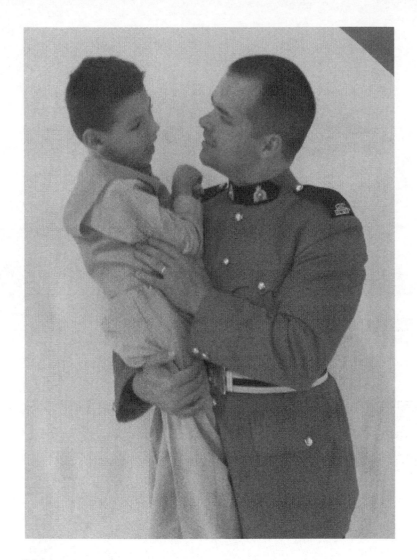

2014

{2012}

Kindergarten graduation

When James was five, he graduated with the kindergarten class at his school. His school days were set up to spend the mornings in the developmental centre, with kids from age 3 to grade 8 with high developmental and physical needs. They worked on gross and fine motor skills, did physiotherapy, and worked on life skills. After lunch he would spend an hour in his grade class, surrounded by peers within the normal schooling system.

James was so accepted within his kindergarten class, and he often came home with piles of pictures and notes from the girls in his class. He's always been a ladies man!

On the day of his graduation I was attending the graduation ceremony. I was filled with excited butterflies as I arrived, and sat in the back behind all of the students, by myself. I was so proud that my boy was graduating kindergarten.

And there he was, proudly sitting straight up in his wheelchair, beside all of his classmates who were seated on risers, waiting for everything to start. They called the students up by last name alphabetically, so James was near the end. One by one they went to get their diploma; some of them ran, some giggled, many stopped to wave at their parents, some were loud, others were silent and shy. They were all so adorable.

Then they called James' name. I could not have looked any prouder. As his aide went to push him across the front of the risers to his teacher to get his diploma, one of the little girls in his class ran over and asked to push him. So there went James, squealing with joy looking back at his little friend who was pushing him, arms drawn into his body, little legs kicked straight out, rolling towards his teacher. And there I am, a sobbing mess, watching him so happy and accepted, passing a milestone that we didn't know if we would see. James squealed with delight as his teacher handed him a diploma, which he promptly crumpled the way that he does, and she placed the guardian angel necklace around his neck.

Seeing him participate in something so normal, without me, fills my heart with a joy that I will never be able to articulate in words. Any special needs mom will understand what I am talking about. I do not get to take for granted what he will be involved in, or accepted into. His programs are set up differently, and for good reason, but we often miss out on the normal milestones, events, and recognitions. He didn't need to be included in this day, as he was in the developmental program, not enrolled in Kindergarten. But people went out of their way to include him, make him feel wanted and accepted, and recognize him the same way that every other child was recognized. I will never take these events for granted; I will treasure deeply each and every one of these kinds of days that my James gets to participate in.

{2013- 2014}

James is a happy, bright, very observant little seven year old. He uses a wheelchair when we are out and in school. He rides the bus home after school in his wheelchair and still uses a car seat in our van. We know that at some point we will need a wheelchair adapted van, but for now he is still too little in our hearts to be riding in a wheelchair everywhere.

He has a rifton activity chair in our home, with an iv pole and feeding pump beside him. Along with his tube feeds, he also eats anything pureed orally. He likes to eat what we are eating, so I will usually make him a plate, show him, and then puree it. He likes to know he's eating what we are eating! His favorite foods are cheesecake, yogurt, grilled cheese with tomato soup and mashed potatoes with gravy.

When he isn't in his activity chair at home, you will find him rolling around on the floor. Rolling into bedrooms, kicking the door closed behind him, and then crying because he is all alone! Or on the couch under a blanket, watching ICarly or Full House.

He loves to paint if you will help him hold the paintbrush, or color if you will help him hold the marker. He loves watching his sister be silly, and is always feeding the dog any and all food that he can convince people to give him. He loves music and people and sunshine and swimming.

Unfortunately at seven years old he no longer wants to be cuddled to sleep. He still will not fall asleep in his own bed, even though the boy has a sleep safe double bed, worth $10,000. It is a fancy hospital bed, allowing it to feel like a normal bed, but having all the safely and medical features of a hospital bed. James still falls asleep in the living room where he can see and hear what is going on, and then we carry him to his bed once he has fallen asleep. Usually three or four times, because if he wakes up when you pick him up or while you are carrying him, you are starting all over again!

James in integrated into grade one for the afternoon at his school, and is in the developmental program in the mornings. He is working on fine motor skills and communication skills in the developmental program.

They have tried using the PECS (picture exchange communication system) with James in school, with limited success. Outside of school, we have also tried this system, with the help of occupational and speech language therapists, with small successes again. With this system, the idea is to be able to pick from a board of several choices of small pictures showing options available. The child is then supposed to pick up the card, and hand it to who is he communicating with, and then he will receive what is on the card that he chose. His fine motor skills are not very precise and they take a lot of work. The only way we found any success within this program was to only offer two choices at a time, and to take away the step of him handing the card back. He is social enough that he will look at the card that he wants, and when you ask if he chose that one, he will acknowledge with a smile and a noise for yes, or a very obvious head shake for a no.

His school began scanning with him early this year, with a great deal of success. They would do this on a smart board, and gave James a big mack button on his wheelchair tray, programmed to say "yes please". Or another communication device, with two large options, one to say "yes please" and one to say "no thank you". When picking songs, they would set the smart board to scan. It would highlight a song, and then continue to move across the board, keeping only one song highlighted at a time. It would then get to the next page icon, and James would say yes. He was able to scan through over twenty pages to find his favorite song every time, Wheels On The Bus.

We worked on doing some scanning on an ipad with him along with his occupational and speech language therapists, with no success. Even with every tool possible, every scanning method, different programs, different selecting styles and methods, his precision just isn't nearly precise enough to be able to communicate effectively on an ipad. It always ended with him feeling so frustrated, which is not what you want when they are learning to communicate.

James attended respite a few times this year, for a week at a time, and he did so good! He was comfortable with the surroundings there, and he knew most of the staff by now. Because he is so socially aware and so cute, everyone always remembers him and comes in to say hi when he is there. He was even friends with the cleaning ladies who came in. He laughed, begged them to take him for walks around the building and outside, and ate well. He also slept well, however, it was never in his bed. He had them all wrapped around his finger! They knew when James was coming, to simply make a bed on the large bean bag in front of the television in the main area by the nurses desk, where he could always see someone if he woke up. On one stay, there was another child who also used the bean bag to sleep at night. So, on the one night that their stays overlapped each other, the nurse actually wheeled James' bed out from his bedroom so he could still sleep in front of the tv too! James would usually give the staff his cutest pouty face at bedtime also, which scored him being rocked to sleep once the other children were tucked in for the night.

He is now 105 cm long, and 42 lbs. When I carry him into his room to lay him in bed, I have to turn very sideways, so I don't hit his head or his feet on the door frame. And lets be honest, this has happened more times than I am willing to admit. He is becoming interested in what we are eating at the table, and enjoys sucking on a piece of steak or farmer sausage. He is very willing to eat what we have eaten, but pureed.

James went to Camp Easter Seal in Watrous Saskatchewan for the first time this year. It was incredible! This camp is dedicated to both children and adults with intellectual and physical disabilities. James was the youngest at his camp, with kids several years older than him. When we pulled up to the camp to drop James off, it was surreal. My heart was beating quite fast, and my eyes couldn't help but tear up. My baby was going to camp; an experience that I didn't think he would ever be given. I unloaded James, and all of his stuff. And wow, was there ever stuff. I had to pack him enough clothes for all week, which is about three times the amount of stuff you would pack for a normal child to attend camp. All of his food, feeding supplies, incontinent supplies, wheelchair, iv pole, medications, bedding, and normal camp supplies. We took him, and all of his supplies, up to his cabin first and got him all setup.

His cabin was all high needs children, and the ratio of campers to cabin leaders was one to one, which was so good for my heart. I was very anxious to leave James with a bunch of very young adults. It felt like I had not given them any information. I had filled out all the forms detailing his feeding and medication schedule, and other than that, they said I could simply go. How was I just supposed to leave him?

So I overstayed my welcome a little bit maybe. I was most definitely that uneasy lurking mom, taking care of all the details that I didn't need to be bothering myself with. I made his bed all cute, like it is at home, even arranging his little pillow and stuffed Eyeore the way he likes them. I set out jammies on the pillow. I set up his diapering supplies, and personally walked the medications down to the nurse. Then I sat with James and his cabin mates and cabin leaders outside for quite a while – I just wasn't ready to leave. James was pretty tearful already, he must have known I was leaving him there. Of course he knew I was leaving him there! I had been talking about it all week!

The young leaders seemed unsure when he would start to cry, and asked how to stop it. As if I had a magical answer, or there was simply a switch I could flip to make it stop. This made me incredibly nervous. I knew how long this boy could cry if he wanted to! I was pretty sure they were going to call me back to pick him up shortly.

I also requested to speak with who would be doing his feedings, so that I could be reassured that they understood his tube feedings, and that they understood what he could and could not eat orally.

Finally, I left. I said my goodbye and bravely walked away, to around the corner, where I stood for a few minutes listening to him cry. So I really wasn't all that brave in my leaving! I stood there until he stopped crying, and I peered back around to see him one more time. He was still on the verge of tears! Stupid! I should have assumed that he was fine and just left. I drove home feeling awful for having left him there.

Thankfully, they allow you to call, and let you know the best times during the day to talk to your child's cabin leaders. So, the next day I called, hoping to hear encouraging news. It wasn't so much encouraging, as it was me apologizing to the young leader. James had cried aaaallllll night. Keeping everyone in the cabin awake. That killed my heart. I volunteered right away to come and pick him up, but they said I should give it more time. So each day I called, and each day the report got a little bit better. By day three he was loving the kids in his cabin and his leaders. He was loving meal times and boat times. By the end of the week he was even sleeping through the night! As long as someone held his hand while he fell asleep, he would sleep! Who's child is this anyway?!

  I picked him up after his five nights away, and he was a happy child! He loved all of his leaders, and I was absolutely blown away by the relationship that he had built with each leader that week. They all came out to my van with us and said their goodbyes, and James laughed and high fived them all good bye. These kids work at this camp all summer, with little to no downtime. Sometimes they get stuck in a cabin with a first time camper with extreme separation anxiety, who cries until he pukes constantly, and keeps everyone else awake all night. They don't get a nap on the basis that their campers did not let them sleep, they simply keep working. But they do this with their summer because this isn't merely a job to them. They are outstanding young adults, with compassion filled hearts, to do the hard things that most people walk away from. They love those among us who many consider to be unlovable. They do their personal hygiene, feeding, showering, diapering, all without complaint and with dignity. They make each camper there feel special and important. There is never an emphasis on what they cannot do. They modify everything and give these children the week of a lifetime. They love in a way that most people do not know how to love. He was clean, well groomed, well fed, rested, and happy.

What a joy to finally have my boy home! Unfortunately, he was miserable for days. This happened after every respite visit also. He got so used to being waited on hand and foot, to having his every demand granted, that he expected the same of me. And that is just not how our home functions.

After three days of this, his attitude wasn't entirely going away yet. He was still yelling at me every time I was in the kitchen, and I could never figure out what he wanted. Eventually I called and spoke with the kitchen at camp to see what they had fed him! She went over the food schedule with me, and told me that everything they made to eat that week was pureed up, and he always ate what everyone else ate. So I went through that menu at home to see what it was that he was wanting. He wanted hot dogs and grilled cheese! At least now I could make those and he finally stopped yelling at me. But let me tell you, pureeing a hot dog, will make you wretch. The texture, the smell. It's a pretty effective deterrent to snacking that's for sure!

James grew up and changed so much this year. He changed drastically both socially and physically. Along with getting longer, bigger, and more socially independent, he got hairier. Seriously, this kid was born a monkey with all of his body hair. And I have always been warned that he will likely hit puberty very early. But the body hair on this kid is unreal! And the body hair where no mother wants to see hair, disturbing. This is only the tip of things that a mother should not have to deal with everyday though, the changes will continue to happen. I just pray that it happens slowly enough that my poor mom heart is not too shocked. It terrifies me to my core to know that while his body is changing, and he is becoming more aware of that, and having no concept of socially acceptable behaviour, that will also be my job to manage. I have worked with disabled adults, so I have seen this handled well, and handled horridly. This is a bridge that I will cross as necessary, and for now, I just keep praying that bridge takes a long long long time to build.

{2014 – 2015}

In August of 2014 we moved from our small college town of Caronport, Saskatchewan to the small northern city of Prince Albert Saskatchewan, as this is where my husband's first posting with the Royal Canadian Mounted Police has taken us. James was the slowest to accept our new home. We bought a nice bungalow style house, which has been nicely redone. Nothing fancy, but welcoming and homey. James has a lovely, clean, fair sized room, and down right refused to sleep in it for the first three weeks that we were there! He would have nothing to do with his new room. If he wasn't in the living room he was crying. And the basement! The evil terrifying basement!! If you took him anywhere near the stairs, he would throw the ugliest tantrum. He was not going into the basement! Our basement is all open and finished, and set up with an office, tv area and lots of toys, but he would have nothing to do with it under any circumstance. After about three weeks he began to feel that this was home, and he slowly began sleeping longer stretches of time in his bed in his own room, and even being content in the basement for short periods of time, as long as every other person in the house was also downstairs. His surroundings need to remain consistent for him to feel safe and content.

He began attending school here in September. I had prepared for the adjustment to be rough and slow. We showed up on the first day and Julia's teacher took her off to her new grade four classroom, and I took James down to his classroom, the developmental education class.

This school is Kindergarten to grade eight, has an English program, French immersion program, and a developmental education program, for children ages 3 to grade 8, with profound physical and intellectual disabilities. From the moment I wheeled him into his new classroom, he loved it. He looked back at me as I left, but never shed a single tear. He loved all of the education assistants immediately and there really didn't seem to be any adjustment period at all. He rode the bus home that day, an hour long bus ride, and loved every second of it.

The classroom has a teacher, around ten educational assistants, and around 20 children. They have their own bus which picks up and drops everyone off at their door. Because this school is out of our district, and we chose to also send Julia there to keep them at the same school, we have to drive her to and from school every day. She is not allowed on the developmental education bus with James. With the bus route, the bus wouldn't pick James up until 9:10am each morning, and Julia starts classes at 8:50 each morning, so I drive them both to school, and pick up only Julia after school. James loves riding the bus so I would never take that away from him.

He sits near the back of the bus, where all of the wheelchairs go. And he knows the bus route. If one child is missing and our bus driver takes a new route to the next home, James is shaking his head in the back and yelling, as if to tell him that he has made a wrong turn! If there is a substitute bus driver for the day, James does not take his eyes off the new driver, making sure they do everything like they are supposed to be doing it.

He comes off the bus tired but happy every day. And completely soaked! His drooling has become uncontrollable. I make fleece bibs that pull over the head for him, as I find they are the most absorbent. But he soaks through them so fast! His bib, shirt and pants or shorts are always soaked through with drool when he gets off the bus. And he has usually peed through his diaper onto his pants, and sometimes the bottom of his shirt. So he's basically a happy, soaking wet, sometimes pee soaked kid by the end of every day.

At his school, a physical therapist regularly comes in to work with the kids, set up equipment, set up programs, and teach one of the educational assistants how to do the daily therapy needed. She stays in contact with the parents, and encourages them to come into the school when she is there to address any concerns that we may be having.

They have a smart board, an amazing snoozlen room, a whirlpool snoozlen room, physio room, many ceiling lifts, tracks, and swings, and open concept boys and girls washrooms with many styles of toilets to allow toileting of each child where it is possible. A snoozlen room is something that is slowly becoming very popular in Canada. Its purpose is to stimulate people who are generally very calm and inattentive, and calm people who tend to be more hyperactive and anxious.

We had never toileted James at home before, but they began putting him on a special tomato toilet seat at school. And while it is lucky to sit him there when he was going to urinate anyways, sometimes he does pee on the potty! And he is so very proud of himself! So we ordered the Rifton HTS toileting system, which will allow us to toilet him safely at home. He was asking us to go potty at home, which is something I had never even considered trying with him. However, he was yelling at me and pointing to go! So one day I held him on our toilet, but he is so skinny and his muscles are so tight, that there is no way to hold him on there in a way that makes him feel safe enough to relax. So nothing happened that night, and we held off until our Rifton arrived.

We now have this chair, and he goes in cycles. Sometimes he would rather just stay in his diaper. Other days he holds his pee and yells at me until I put him on the Rifton, and he goes immediately! It amazes me what he is able to accomplish as the years go by. I think sometimes I get so stuck in routine that I forget that he is always slowly advancing.

The school takes the kids on outings several times a week. Every Tuesday they all go to the gymnastics club and play for an hour and a half in the morning. On Fridays half of the class goes bowling, and they alternate. They take shopping trips often for supplies for the class and take a few kids with. They go outside to play and do activities regularly with their grade eight buddies.

Daily Routine {2015}

As I am writing this, James is three months shy of turning eight. Our daily routine with James looks like this during the school year:
6:45 – Wake James. Although who are we really kidding here! Usually he has been up for hours and is either happily but loudly talking in his bed, or I had crawled into his bed hours earlier to try to save everyone's sleep from his middle of the night yelling.
6:50 – Change diaper, carry from bed to Rifton Activity chair in living room, strap in. Open the curtains and turn on the tv to family channel.
6:55 – Prepare pump with pump kit, water, and formula for both breakfast and lunch. Hook pump feed up to James.

7:00 – Prepare and feed James orally for breakfast. Always baby cereal mixed with whole milk, and a yogurt.

7:10 – Basic grooming. Wash face. Check ears, hands, brush hair and teeth.

7:15 – Pack both kids lunches. For James I set out a pureed lunch – soup, homemade food, with a yogurt or a pudding.

7:30 – Get myself ready

7:45 – Turn off James' pump feed. Disconnect feed, flush extension. Prep formula feed for lunch at school (I only need to add a little extra water). Pack pump, extension, and oral lunch into lunch kit. Leave James in his chair as long as possible to digest. The sooner I lie him down the higher the risk of vomiting.

8:10 – Lift James from Rifton chair to the floor, always having a blanket in case he vomits. Get his diaper changed and get him dressed – this can take five minutes or fifteen minutes depending on how stiff he is. Make sure any tender spots on his feet are bandaged and covered by socks and shoes (he kicks very hard all of the time so I am very diligent in trying to avoid skin breakdown). Add a bib to the outfit so he isn't drool soaked by the time we get to school.

8:25 – Carry James from floor in living room to van. Secure in car seat. Add backpack to back of wheelchair, making sure the wheelchair pack also has the necessary supplies in it.

8:30 – Drive both kids to school.

8:40 – Drop off Julia. Lift 55lb wheelchair out of van. Lift James into wheelchair, and wheel him into his class.

8:45 – FREEDOM

3:45 – James returns home on the bus. Carry James inside, load wheelchair into the back of the van. Get James' diaper changed or toilet him, clothes changed, and lift him into his Rifton chair by the window – where he likes to sit until supper.

4:00 – Unpack his backpack. Throw away pump bag, attach pump to pump stand, and load with a new kit for the morning.

5:00 – Supper. Feed James orally a pureed meal, with a yogurt or pudding or cheesecake. Syringe a blended homemade whole foods formula into his Mic-key button – about 10 – 35ml syringes, given slowly over an hour. Plus one or two syringes of whole milk, and two more of water.

6:30 – Change diaper or toilet. Bath. Bathing involves lifting him into the tub, bathing him, lifting him out wet as safely as possible. Drying, dressing in pyjamas, and carrying back out of the bathroom. It usually leaves me exhausted.

7:00 – Feed James his oral snack, always baby cereal mixed with whole milk, and a yogurt if he wants more. Prepare and administer medications by g-tube.

8:10 – Change diaper, change pyjamas if he has gotten them dirty. Lie on couch where I have to lie beside him until he falls asleep.

9 – Midnight – Move James into his bed once he is in a deep enough sleep.

Each day his outfit is changed two to six times depending on how many times he pees out of a diaper, throws up, and how badly he is drooling. We go through ten to fifteen bibs a day, and five to ten receiving blankets a day. Plus anything else that he manages to puke on.

This schedule is only what I do directly with him. It doesn't include what I need to do daily to prepare for James' care, what I need to do with my ten year old daughter, family things, and housework.

Medical supplies need to be kept stocked up and ordered regularly as everything needs to be ordered in. Ordering and pickup is all done while the kids are in school. His blended formula is all homemade, and every ingredient needs to be cooked before being put into the formula as he doesn't digest raw ingredients well. Every ingredient is cooked, pureed in the magic bullet, put through the blender, and then made into a mix. Then all the dishes are done by hand. All of his oral feeds are homemade with high healthy fats added to everything. I do large batches every few days and freeze small portions, so he gets several flavor combinations and nutrients at every meal. Even his desserts are homemade with high fats.

While at home James likes to be in his rifton activity chair at the window, watching people walk and drive by. He also likes to be in the kitchen if I am cooking or doing dishes. If Julia is upstairs he enjoys being on the floor to follow her around the house, being a pretty typical bratty little brother.

A lot of our communication with specialists is done during business hours, while the kids are in school. Often carpets or furniture needs to be cleaned from vomit. Laundry is never ending.

Our house is only 1000 sq ft, and it is being overtaken with equipment! Along with a rifton activity chair we also have a rifton hts commode, iv pole, bath chair, rifton walker, double size sleep safe bad, and endless medical and feeding supplies in the house. In the garage and the van, we keep his tilt in space wheelchair, the convaid cruiser chair, and the special tomato pushchair. We also have a recliner both upstairs and downstairs that he sits safely in as long as someone is in the room. He gets around by rolling on the floor still, so I vacuum every day, as we have a burnese mountain dog in the house.

Taking James on outings in the summer is quite easy, but I see this winter becoming more challenging. I can still very awkwardly change him in the van in summer, but once winter comes it will get a little tricky again. Some malls are redoing family bathrooms which often include a couch, which works perfectly for us as I can safely and comfortably lie him on there, with privacy, to change him.

Baby change tables are becoming quite dangerous with how long and stiff he is. I did think far enough ahead to order the portable kit and bag with our Rifton HTS chair, allowing us to put a stand and the seat of the commode into a very large bag, lug it with into a public bathroom, set it up over a public toilet, and allow him to use the toilet. However, this does me no good if I am by myself and still have to try to figure out how to get a diaper on and off of him safely and well in that transition! I'm sure I will learn that magic when the time comes, right?!

This was a great year for James' overall. It was a hard year for me. I started working two jobs casually that I really loved. One with high needs adults, and one in a high school cafeteria. I think I have pretty much lost both of those now though. James was on and off sick all this year, with a few months involving random high fevers with no explanation. The fevers were followed by a very lethargic sick day, and then back to normal the next day. We never did find a cause.

His vomiting was out of control for many months, mostly beginning in January. Any time I would mention this to one of our specialists, they would hear me out, see the weight loss that was happening, and encourage me to up his formula intake. He needed more calories. However, I firmly believe that after almost six years of formula intake, his stomach was starting to reject it.

Can you imagine being formula fed every single day? I can't imagine it provides much energy, and it can't feel very good to digest. And his puke smelt so badly; like sickly sweet. It was nauseating!

So, without any help, I began to switch up his diet. I upped what he ate by mouth, adding more fats. Adding fat to everything I could without making things too rich – too much fat makes him puke. And I began to experiment with blended foods going straight into his g-tube. It was a long six months of trial and error, and we still aren't fully switched, nor do I have it all figured out, but for the first time in years, he gained weight! He went from 42 pounds, to 47.5 pounds. Finally!

So while I am pretty sure that I lost the two jobs that I thought I could fit into my schedule, I have realized that I am still needed just at home. Just. I make it sound like it is nothing. It feels like nothing so often when people ask what I do with all of my time. I don't feel like I have much time! So much of my life is always revolving around what James needs, and that is something that I can't explain very well to someone who hasn't walked in these shoes. So for the next year, I am going to try to be content enough to just be the mom that I am needed to be. Even though to everyone else, it seems that I am living the life, with loads of time for only me. If only I could tell them.

We are coming to the end of our summer vacation now, and the kids both go back to school in three weeks. And my friends are either heading back to their jobs at the same time as their children, or have been working through the summer. And I dread the typical, "oh I wish that I could be home like you" that always comes with this time of year. When they ask what I did that first week that they are back in school, and my response is "I slept", I dread the guilt that I feel, the uselessness that I feel, and the comments about how nice it must be to have my days free and to myself.

And I won't correct any of those comments. I am lucky to be able to be home. I am beyond thankful that I am able to be home and do what is needed. But please know, that someone who is a full time caregiver to a completely dependent child, is not sitting on the couch all day with their feet up watching their stories. There are times where things are going smoothly and I do get that time! Absolutely! But most of the time my days are consumed, whether he is home with me or in school, with his care.

Now that I have gone slightly sideways, I will get back to the year in general. It ended well. I have decided to stay home this year and not pursue outside jobs – we will see if this actually happens. It's so completely against my nature! James gained weight for the first time in years. Everyone is adjusted to our new city and their new classrooms, and we are ready to take on the next year.

Will There Be Healing?

When James was very young, starting around the three month mark, we began to struggle with peoples responses to James' "illness", and their views on healing. Once we had that first CT scan done, and I was no longer the crazy paranoid mom who was dreaming up ridiculous issues that didn't actually exist, people started to feel that they had the freedom to impose all kinds of crazy on us.

We are a Christian family, and believe wholly that our God can heal. I believe that He has healed many in the past, and that presently He still heals. I believe in healing miracles. But we do not agree with many of the things that we experienced when James was so young, and we were so fragile and vulnerable.

I was so afraid for my baby, of all the unknowns, of losing him completely, of him living a tortured life, feeling pain that he couldn't even tell me about. My pregnancy had been so perfect; I felt like I'd been flung into this so unprepared. My heart had no time to process that I didn't go into the hospital, and come home with a perfect little healthy baby. Our lives were not continuing as they were supposed to. I felt so very alone. No one really knows what a mother feels during this time, except another mom who has walked the same road. And I didn't have anyone like that to lean on. I was surviving.

We were invited to a house church one Sunday around James' four month mark. We had never been before, so we weren't entirely sure what to expect. We arrived and expected to sit quietly and take it all in, see what it was all about. I am very much an introvert, and that together with my sheer exhaustion, was about all I could handle. Unfortunately, that is so far from what happened.

They were going to pray for healing for James. Straight out for healing. No in between. No practical help for the family. No peace and rest and wisdom for the medical professionals that we were working with. No comfort and sleep for James. We were asked just before they started if this was ok, and like a deer in the headlights I shook my head yes. I wanted to crawl out of my skin. Scream. Cry. Some warning should have been given. We should have known what we were walking into.

This probably sounds dramatic. After all, a nice Christian group of people wants to pray for your baby, for healing, which obviously is all your own heart desires, and I'm saying that I wanted to run. Why wasn't I overcome with thankfulness? Did I not have enough faith? I struggled with this. People told me that I didn't have enough faith in the healing, or it would have happened. Did I really not have enough faith? Was I failing somewhere in my spiritual walk?

I think that there is a place for this. I think that it was very appropriate for people to come alongside us, when we were exhausted and scared and running on empty, and to hold up the things that we couldn't. I was only surviving. I needed people to hold James up in prayer in a way that my heart couldn't.

Why couldn't my heart ask, without hesitation and with full belief that it would happen, for that complete healing? That is all I wanted, it was my hearts true desire. The answer is simple; because I was James' mom. I was the one up all night, every night. I was the one who walked a screaming baby for hours on end, while taking care of a toddler, making meals and cleaning the house. I was the one who went to every specialist appointment and received every test result. I was the one who saw the damage done to his tiny little brain. I was the one who held his tiny body tightly as it violently tremored every single night. And I was the one who was going to continue doing this every single night on almost zero sleep, without an end in sight. While I hoped that a miracle would happen, and my heart was so open to that, I also had to guard my heart. I had to stay in touch with my current reality; I had to be able to keep going. I had to keep putting one foot in front of the other, when absolutely no hope or help was anywhere in sight.

So, back to that Sunday morning. We sat in the middle of a circle of people, who prayed for James' healing, for over an hour. I was far too exhausted to sit there for an hour, while people prayed prayers five and ten minutes long each. I felt so unsettled. It terrified me. Most of these people I had never even met before. We did not ask for this, and did not receive adequate warning that this was going to be happening. My skin tingled, I felt dizzy. I was not hearing the words; I was clutching James and praying we could leave. I cried while people prayed. Not because I was touched by the words, but because I couldn't handle or process what was happening.

What happened that morning changed nothing. James remained the same. We did not continue to go to that house church. However, after taking a few Sundays off from that church all together, we did continue to go to the main service. These people tried to do what they felt was right, and with pure intentions. However, it was just done wrong. It felt like a slap in the face. If that had happened to us today, I would be much better equipped to deal with it. I would not have allowed it to happen in the same way again. But I do know that the hurt that they caused, was not intentional. Some of those people became a huge part of our early years raising James.

One day I had a friend call me; she had heard that James was sick. It was out of genuine care and concern, she just maybe had never been in such a situation before. One of her comments stayed with me for years, " What sin do you have in your life that James was born this way." If I were being honest, that hurt me for years. Seven to be exact. I did not tell her until James was seven years old that her comment had hurt so deeply. And when I told her, she was devastated that I hadn't told her earlier. She didn't even remember saying it.

I've learnt that so many people have never been in situations like this in their lifetime. They have not been around someone who is disabled, yet still led a quality life and was loved everyday simply for who they are. Until recently, it was common for families to give up children born with a disability and adults who acquired one later on. They lived their lives in institutions while the families continued on with their normal lives. That doesn't happen as much any longer. We are realizing that these people are gifts! They teach us far more about love and quality of life that we ever could have dreamed.

This friend was not the only person who relayed the message to me that James' illness was a direct reflection of the sin in my life. NO. Sickness, all sickness, I believe is a direct reflection of the sin in the world today. Everything that causes disabilities and sickness', mankind has created. We are all a part of that. I've sat through sermons and public speakers, stating very similar things; James was the punishment for my sin. This simply is not the case, and my heart will not allow this in.

I had people email me when they heard about healing revivals happening in churches, and then follow up with "why aren't you taking James? Do you not want him to be healed? Do you not believe?" I had people calling me suggesting new healing doctors and therapies. I tried to deal with everyone graciously, but I'm not sure that my tone was always that gracious.

I've heard so many different things regarding healing, and why James was or wasn't healed. When you read the gospels, we see Jesus healing so many! However, while He heals many, He also steps over many who need healing, not choosing them, to heal others. Why? Can we ever really know why? I don't think so. Someone suggested that because Jesus could foresee their lives, he chose not to heal them because of the things they would do. I do not agree with this either. That would be like telling me that if James would have been healed, he would do horrible things, so God decided that he would be in a wheelchair, non verbal, tube fed, diapered, and struggle in so many areas of life, simply to take away his free will.

James was never healed completely. His brain damage is still present. I do believe that God can choose to miraculously heal James at any moment that he wishes to do so. However, I also know that James' healing may come when he goes to Heaven. When he will run and sing with all the children. When his body won't hurt and fight against him.

While he was not healed, James is a miracle. In June 2010, James went for his second CT scan, and this was a miracle in itself. He had the scan, and we returned to Royal University Hospital in Saskatoon the following week to meet with the neurologist for the results. We would see a new neurologist this time, since James' other one had since retired. This would be the first time he would have met James.

After waiting in the office for a while, the neurologist entered the room. He looked at James, who was lying on the table in the room on his back, looking around. When the door opened he startled and looked to see who was coming in. The doctors eyebrows crinkled, like he was confused, and his gaze moved to me. He checked the chart, confirmed that this was James, and then moved over to him on the table. He began a head to toe examination quickly of James, testing his reflexes, and looking puzzled, all while interacting with James. Once he was done he asked us to join him in the next room to see the results of the scan ourselves.

We followed him into a tiny room next door with computer monitors displaying dozens of images. He asked us both to take a seat, and James sat in his stroller behind us. He then started talking.

He asked if I had noticed the funny look he was giving us in the other office, and I said that I had! How could I not notice? He said that he had just read the scan results before entering our room, and was expecting to find a little boy, in a very vegetative state. He should not have been able to move much, his eyes should not have been able to make contact, nor should he be able to recognize people and make connections that way. He should not have understood anything enough or had any personal connections to the outside world which would initiate a smile.

Yet, there was James, kicking, smiling, laughing, and very clearly seeing and understanding that someone new had just walked into the room. A boy who knew who mom and dad were, and who was capable of very strong ties and loving relationships. None of this should have been possible with the level of brain damage that he was seeing on the images. James brain was less than half the size of what it should be, and what was there was littered with cysts and calcifications. He had no medical reasoning for why James was able to make eye contact with us. For why James actually knew us. For why James was capable of developing trusting and loving relationships. For why James was so observant and aware of the world around him.

I cried after that appointment. James may not have been healed to the standard that other people had hoped for, but he was healed! He was capable of love and trust, and that was going to increase his quality of life far beyond what we had initially prepared for.

The issue of healing when you are dealing with a child with severe and profound disabilities is something that each heart has to decide for itself. For me it took time to be open to possibilities.

I do not believe in my heart that any hurt was ever meant when this topic was brought to my attention by many people. But I would like to pass on some suggestions to people who have never been in this situation, but who may find themselves in someone's life who will face these scenarios.

My first suggestion would be love. Approach the person with love. Remember that you are dealing with people, with hearts, not with a situation. Please, make eye contact, be sensitive to how they are feeling, let them lead the conversation. Do not go "cold turkey". Their hearts are fragile and hurting, lost, scared. This is not a good time for you to do something for on looking people to think you have your spiritual life all together. Lead with love.

Meet a practical need during your journey with them. Whether that is making them a meal, watching their children for two hours, stopping to ask them how they are doing and actually listening, bringing over some hot fresh buns. By taking the time to meet a practical need you will get a glimpse into their reality that they might not have shared with you otherwise.

Be understanding if any attempt you make to pray for their child, or them, or anything else, is turned down, or even accepted with limits. Their hearts have to be ready; they have to have a grasp on what they are dealing with, what they believe, and they have to want what you are offering. Pushing anything can cause hurt like you cannot imagine.

    Being a Christian, surrounded by Christians, and watching others go through medical trials can be a struggle. I say this having recently watched several people I know give birth to either babies with known health complications, or very early births where they needed a little extra help in the NICU to get up and going. Watching these families ask for prayer for specific concerns, and seeing each day that these requests are being fulfilled as requested, followed by endless comments such as: "God is good," "God will take care of your baby because he loves your baby," "Keep trusting and everything will work out," "God is faithful to his children," can cut quite deeply. I am not saying that these things should not be said, because I too have said them. But they sting for so many families. James wasn't healed. We thought we were having a perfectly healthy baby. We loved God. A child being sick is never the will of our God. A child struggling is never the will of God. A child having to fight every single day to breathe without aspirating, to swallow food, to make their hand move, to keep still and sleep, is never the will of God. It is never the result of lack of faith, lack of prayer, lack of trust. It is never the outcome from being loved less by their creator. Their creator hurts with them, and with their families, and he longs for the day he will make that tiny body perfect. We may never see that on this side of Heaven; something that breaks my heart every single day. Every day I kiss James' forehead, and wish so badly that he could do everything that he wants to do.

Invisible
{2013}

I have become the invisible mom. It doesn't seem to matter what crowd I'm in, I am still the invisible mom. James attends a school with a special needs wing, where he is pretty much a celebrity! Anywhere else we go, I am invisible. I take him to my daughter's school for her parent teacher interviews, concerts, awards, and book fairs. When I am pushing that chair, it seems that I don't exist. And I've become quite accustomed to that. So when that one person comes out of their group of friends, to acknowledge me, or even heaven forbid, have a normal conversation with me, I often look like a deer in the headlights for the first minute. Whatever you have just said to me I most likely did not even hear. I am finding my way out of my "I am just fine" mask, which I wear every time I have to walk through that crowd of laughing moms. Then I realize that I am blowing my only real conversational opportunity, and rush to gather my thoughts and feelings and emotions, and try to respond in a normal and pleasant manner. Often times I tear up. You could ask me if you could borrow my lawn mower, and chances are my eyes will glaze over embarrassingly in the process of answering you, because I am not used to being approached like a normal mom when I am with James.

I walk through crowds of people I know, often people I would call my friends, and feel a desperate aching kind of lonely. They are standing in a circle, kids running around them screaming and laughing, or hanging on a parents arm displaying a full blown temper tantrum. The circle is fairly tight, and a few of them always catch my eye. Yes, I am usually looking, because every single time I know I'm going to be faced with this situation, I vow to not pull away. To not look down the entire time, like my heart is so ready to please just finally do. The few who catch my eye often just glance away. Sometimes I may get a slight acknowledgement by a head nod, or slight smile. But no one moves. Not even slightly to let me in. Nobody even slightly angles out to even hint at politely welcoming me into the circle. It might be awkward if I joined. What would I do with the wheelchair? What if James chokes and causes a scene? What if I am anything but perfect and heaven forbid I am even a touch honest about that?

I'm not only invisible in a large crowd scene. I've become invisible with smaller groups of close friends. I went out for supper just a few weeks ago with two other couples with infants and toddlers. The infants joined us for the supper, and the toddler, and my two children were with sitters. The girls sat at one end of the table and the guys at the other, the two babies floating around for everyone to play with and ogle over. These two girls were my friends. People I love and trust. And yes, I became invisible.

What did the evening consist of? Infant milestones, and how the toddler is now interacting with the baby. I sat, and listened with that smile on my face that I have become so unnervingly good at. But I had nothing to add to the conversation. My stories are all different. And not what new moms want to talk about. Ever. Sometimes I have a heart moment with someone who really listens to a story I have about James, about his interactions with his sister, about how hard it is for Julia to be the big sister. I could count those moments for you they are so few and far between. So as our night went on, my heart broke, over and over and over. Not because I am jealous. Because not only am I hearing again and again how different James is, my heart is hearing over and over again how different I have become. I wouldn't change who I have become through this, but I have become painfully aware that I just don't fit anymore. I try every single day, and it is so draining.

  I am the invisible mom that everyone knows, and everyone sees. But I'm much easier to pass by than to welcome in. I spend my time and my energy shielding James from just this. Does he know that he is different? Does he know how different he is? Is he seeing the 99 people that have turned away when he makes eye contact with them? Or does he hang onto that one person who held his gaze, and maybe even returned it with a smile. I get so angry when I see him ignored. Dammit people, I love your kids. Your kids who are running around with stinky breath, being disobedient and rude and obnoxious, with snot rolling down their face like Niagara Falls. I take the time to smile at them, say hi, acknowledge their new outfit or toy or bike riding skills. I don't look away when they look into my eyes. When they talk to me I listen. James may not talk, but he squeals with delight, and if you'd take the ten seconds with him to invoke this, you will remember it forever. He is genuine and delightful and so full of unconditional love. And when you choose to ignore him, you also ignore me. When his heart breaks my heart breaks. And right now his heart doesn't appear to break very often, but mine breaks every time that I know his heart should have broken. His innocence is still protecting him, and I pray that he holds onto this for as long as humanly possible.

  This is my battle every single time we go out. My love for James and my family is what holds my heart together. I know that I am going to be invisible. That my heart is going to break. That I am going to be on display.

That people are always watching me. Celebrities complain about the paparazzi. The world is my paparazzi. I am always being judged on how I handle James. Sometimes I am admired, and those moments I hang onto. I could tell you each time that I felt that when caring for James in a public setting, because they are so rare. People don't look me in the eye, but they are watching how I react to James' outbursts. They are disgusted that I simply reach over to wipe drool off his face with his bib while in the midst of a conversation or during a meal. They are disgusted when I search for a place to change his diaper in a public washroom. I'd like to know if they have a better solution to the problem of him needing to be changed.

This will always be one of the hardest topics for me to talk about. I chose very young in James' life, that while I had him, I would not make work outside of the home my priority; he would be my priority. My life would be given meaning through the care I would give him, the purpose that I would allow his life to have would fulfill my purpose. I just never knew that this was an impossibly lonely road.

{2015} My husband has become a Royal Canadian Mounted Police officer since I began this book. We now live in Prince Albert, Saskatchewan, and have been here for just over six months. And I am the loneliest that I have ever been. I have a few acquaintances through the church that we found here, but people are very busy in their lives. And I don't have the freedom that I desire to go and pour into other people's lives. I am not a surface person, I never have been. I wear my heart on the outside and I look for deep relationships.

However, having felt like an invisible mom for seven years, I have to fight everyday to stay true to myself. I face far more rejection once people see into my life than I do acceptance, and I've started to put up walls that are getting harder to break down.

Our outings have gotten harder and I feel on display more than ever. James is forty five pounds now, still in a car seat, and I still lift his fifty plus pounds wheelchair into the back of the van. He is 110cm tall, so I look ridiculous carrying him, as I am only 5'3". He thinks it is hilarious to squirm away from me and fight against me as I buckle him into his wheelchair, so that is usually quite the gong show. Then once we are inside our destination, he is either incredibly happy and loud, or incredibly angry and loud!

Thank you to those people who take the time to make eye contact with James, touch his hand, say hi to him. Thank you to those people who acknowledge me behind the wheelchair, often pulling a shopping cart behind me. Thank you for taking a second to hold a door for me, or pass me the shoe that James kicked off, or simply smile to say you see me. It means the world to me. Often people with disabilities say that they feel invisible when they go out. Let me tell you that the caregivers often feel invisible too.

James has given my life a purpose that I had never dreamed. However, I am still Dawn. I am still that girl who loves to laugh and have fun and go out alone and with friends. Sometimes I dream of working a job that brings home a paycheck and receives recognition for what I have accomplished. I dream of leaving my children with someone to go away with my husband for a week. Or heck, how about a weekend? I dream about sleeping deeply, not needing to keep one ear listening for any sign that James may need me. I dream of going out with friends for supper, or a movie, without rigid deadlines of when I need to be home. Or, where we are living now, I just dream of a friend that isn't an hour and a half drive away. Someone to talk to honestly, and laugh with, and just be me with.

Blog Entry {February 11, 2011} Joy in the Loneliness

Today, as I wondered how to lift the heaviness from my heart, I have decided to let it be. To find a quiet contentment, while getting through the day to day.

My heart has been incredibly heavy lately, comparable to when James was younger, and we were just learning of the struggles that he would face as he grew up. I dropped Julia off at school this morning, and drove the 20 minutes to James' school to drop him off, listening to him "talk" to the sun all the way there from the back seat. James attends a school for high special needs children. Upon entering the first set of doors, was a boy, 14 years old, who is mobile, non verbal, and quite violent. With three adults holding him back, James and I snuck by, and got him settled into his wheelchair. I struggle daily to find the balance between cherishing the present, and looking towards our future. When James was younger, it was so hard to share my heart with others. His differences were so evident to me, but not easily seen by others. He turned 3 in October, and things are much more evident now. All the babies that I held when he was one, are now walking and talking and running and playing. They are eating meals with their families. They are running and playing with their friends. They are learning to communicate what they want and need. They are potty training. They sleep. I am not sad because I wish that James were different. This little boy is such a blessing, and continues to bless me and teach me so much everyday! What I don't talk about is the loneliness that comes with all of this. People have often made comments to me about not coming out to group settings, young moms groups, big groups of girl friends going for coffee. The list goes on. Having a 3.5 year old, who is at a 4-6 month level, and no family around to help, and friends who all have young children that are developing very normally, makes sharing incredibly difficult. I often can't relate, and they can't relate to my heart either.

I've been struggling with the loneliness constantly. And yet, in that loneliness, I am learning to be content. Baby steps! I am daily giving my heart to Jesus. I am much more able to gracefully accept the tears, and keep on going. This morning, after dropping James off at school, I picked myself up a coffee, and went for a walk in Crescent Park. It was only -2 today, -9 with the wind.... but that is still cold enough to freeze tears (I recommend crying indoors when the temp is below 0!!). 3.5 years in I am still learning that it is okay to step back when I need to. Take the tears as they come, and soak up the joy in the small things! Julia drew a picture the other morning. It was her and James, holding hands, walking up a hill pulling a sled, to slide down together. "This is what I will do with James if his cerebral palsy goes away mom".

James' pump is beeping, so I am off to unhook his feed, and do the "mom things"!!

Lamentations 3:22,23 "Because of the Lord's great love we are not consumed for his compassions never fail. They are new every morning; great is your faithfulness."

I dream of not being lonely. However, I know I will always be lonely; my heart is adjusting, and I am usually good with that. This doesn't mean that I've given up. It means I've accepted it, and I look for the smaller displays of love that come my way. I've chosen to remain open and honest, and take the hurt with the joy. I've chosen to pursue things that I love while I am on this journey. My commitment to commit myself to James' quality of life does not mean that I am not still my own person. What brings me joy has just needed to shift to things that I can do alone. I sew beautiful quilts that we cuddle with on the couch. I play my keyboard, usually when it's only me and the kids at home, to spare anyone else's ears from the horrors! I paint and write. I love to cook and bake. I love to look for beautiful things in nature. I love to be outside as much as I can when I get time to myself. I love fresh air and hiking and walking with my feet in a lake. I love horses, but I am terribly allergic, so I love them from far away!

Sometimes if you ask how I am, and I was truly honest with you, my answer would be quiet. I am quiet. Things around me are calm, taken care of, happy. But I'm needing some noise. Not actual noise though, because I like quiet! But my heart is ready for acceptance and real friendship. And don't get me wrong, I have a best friend who shares my heart, and we talk every single day! And she only lives an hour and a half from me ☺ I am missing the everyday, adult relationships.

James is nearing eight years old right now, and the loneliness continues. I used to think that as he got older, this would get easier, because differences become less evident once the ages where children are constantly meeting milestones start to pass. I think I was wrong though. Now I have a huge child that I need to diaper, spoon feed, pump feed, and lift. While other families worry about their child acting out at someone else's' dinner table, I worry about James projectile vomiting all over someone else's dinner table, or pooping while everyone is eating. Because trust me, anytime it is not a good time to do so, he has a bowel movement. And it is anything from discreet. It is the most awkward, uncomfortable situation for everyone involved. And he is eight so it isn't easily hidden, and neither is that smell!

As he continues to get older, that gap between me and parents that I started this journey with, only widens. Our life goals are so different. Our holidays look so different. Our daily schedules are so different. What takes them a half an hour a day to do as a parent, takes me the majority of our waking hours. His hygienic needs are going to be more and more involved, the bigger and older that he gets. Our friends will become empty nesters. They will watch their children go off to university, get married, bring home grand babies. I will be lifting an adult. Diapering an adult. Feeding an adult. Cleansing an adult. The loneliness won't go away.

Mothers Day
{May 12, 2013}

Today is Mother's Day. It is on a Sunday this year and I chose to stay home with my kids today. We cuddled, watched Cheaper by the Dozen one AND two, ate muffins and nachos, and jumped on the trampoline. Later today we are going to a greenhouse and out for lunch.

Sunday mornings for our family usually mean getting up and going to church. However, less and less will you find me in my regular pew on holiday weekends. Or out for supper. Or at bigger events. Why? It is another reminder that I just do not fit anymore. I realize that to many people, that statement alone sounds like an all too familiar pity grab. I assure you it is not. Sit down and listen to the heart of a special needs mom. The deep, honest, raw heart of how our lives and hearts have changed.

I hooked James up to his pump for lunch. His chair was in the livingroom as we were all watching a movie. An hour later it beeped, and I disconnected him. Well, I was going to disconnect him. As I went to lock the extension he began to laugh at me, which is never a good sign! Then I noticed that the extension was actually hanging between his body and the arm of the chair, hanging down towards the carpet where I could not see it. He had disconnected it! My carpet, my ugly blue living room carpet, was absolutely soaked right through, with vanilla pediasure.

Disgusting. I would generally just laugh this off; situations like this are almost daily with James! Today I sat and cried. My heart was tired. I read everyone's mothers day posts with joy for them. I look at their pictures and smiled. And secretly, my heart aches to hear James say "I love you mommy", or "thank you". I want to run and play with both my children. We don't let James' wheelchair keep us from doing things. We run with his chair to keep up, carry him up flights of stairs, carry his body where his chair won't go. I want Julia and James to play on a playground together, get into trouble together, fight, laugh, build forts; the list could go on forever.

I don't raise my children knowing that "this is only a phase." It may be a phase with Julia. Most things are not a phase with James, they are forever. Or, they are going to progressively get harder. James will not outgrow diapers, we will simply find bigger ones. We are limited to where we can go in the winter. He barely fits onto a traditional change table at six years old. And then there's the fact that he is a six year old boy in a women's washroom. I never change him in a public washroom without stares of judgement. What do I do when he no longer fits onto that tiny baby change table? We eat out in restaurants, knowing that if he begins to have a bowel movement, I will spend the rest of the meal time in the van with him, and my leftovers will be brought out to me. We are prepared with blankets and wipes, ready to pull out and catch cupfuls of projective vomit at any moment, which also comes with harsh stares. I am always thankful when one person is kind enough to not look at me judgingly. He will not put himself to sleep, and someday I will not be able to carry him to bed every night. I am barely able to lift his tiny wet naked body out of the bathtub after a bath, at six years old.

What am I going to do when he is ten? When he needs that bath every single day.

He is six years old, with pubic hair. Children with CMV hit puberty very early. I change his diaper, and have to deal with getting a diaper back onto my son, with an erection. Most parents see this when their child is a baby, and they laugh because it is funny! This is my reality, forever. Something that generally never crosses a mothers mind. I spray his nose several times a day with a mild saline, and then clean his nose out. Gross? Absolutely. But just another thing that James cannot do on his own. I do these things every single day for him, because I want people to see the amazingly handsome little boy that he is. But don't think for a second that all of that just happens. If I forget to clip his finger nails he scratches his face or the inside of his mouth or his eyes. If I forget his toe nails he cracks them right to the nail bed by kicking things so hard and his nails hitting first. He doesn't feel pain, so he bites his fingers and hands until they bleed. His legs have massive bruises all the time from kicking hard surfaces and not feeling it. His spine bruises and tears and bleeds and calluses' because he pushes himself around on his back, and he is so thin that those bones stick out so far. We check them daily and do our very best to balance protecting them and letting him be as independent as possible, doing what little boys like to do. He doesn't have control over external or internal muscles in his body. His anus does not always close the way ours does, therefore, he is often quite literally leaking a fecal smell. I work tirelessly everyday to ensure that he is as clean as possible, clothes and diapers changed regularly, and creams applied to minimize the smell so that other people do not notice. He is my son, and I long to see people simply love him. And I work around the clock to make this as much of a reality as possible.

As I mentioned earlier, the later part of our day was going to consist of buying some flowers at a greenhouse and getting some ice cream. We did just that! Julia and I picked out some beautiful lilies, some potting soil, new plants, and a few packages of things to grow from seed. Julia pushed her brother through the greenhouse in his wheelchair. James squealed with delight and kind people stopped to watch Julia take care of her little brother and hold doors open for him. We went for ice cream after, where James devoured a small soft serve sundae and laughed loudly at his sister dipping her French fries into her vanilla ice cream cone.

I do not tell you about how much work James can be to give you the impression that our life is restricted and burdened. Quite the contrary. Our life is full of love and compassion and laughter. Our hearts are always burdened by everything above, in a light kind of way. Everything is taken in stride, in the moment, and we thank God for every day that we are given together. My Mother's Day felt lonely, and my heart was heavy with everything mentioned earlier. And I can still honestly say, this was the best Mother's Day so far. I love my children. Everything above is simply routine for me.

Taking the time to realize why my heart is feeling heavy is all part of the process; it is not the end of the process. I read something on facebook one day, one of those really annoying cartoon type pictures with a caption that they seem to have for absolutely everything insignificant in life! But this one stuck with me. It read, "Feel what you feel, until you feel something different." I've learnt to be in the moment that I'm in, in the emotion, and to stay there until I'm ready to leave.

Taking a Step Back
{2009}

For the first two years of James life, I was constantly overwhelmed with medical appointments. We lived two hours away from where the majority of our medical appointments were, and in those first two years, we were there almost every single week. My husband was a full time student, so I would pack up James, all his equipment, and Julia, and drive from MooseJaw to Saskatoon. We would stay with my parents for a night to make the driving a little easier on the kids. We went back for neonatology appointments, paediatrician, physical therapy, occupational therapy, speech therapy, dietician, feeding clinics, nutrition clinics, neurology, vision tests, hearing tests, swallowing tests, CT scans, MRI's, EEG's, an ng placement, G-tube placement, orthopaedic surgeon, and the list goes on.

Our neonatology appointments ended after the first six months, leaving us in the very capable hands of our developmental paediatrician at the Kinsmen Children's Center. Our various therapists were seeing James every two to three weeks, with hours of stretches and exercised prescribed to do daily at home. I did this faithfully, taking home almost every piece of equipment they thought might help his posture, eating, playing, comfort, fine and gross motor skills. I was beyond exhausted.

Bottle feeding turned into a living nightmare that wouldn't end. James had chest infection on top of pneumonia; he was almost consistently on antibiotics from 12 – 23 months of age. Our dieticians and feeding consultants recommended every possible way to feed him, every possible bottle, different formulas and different levels of thickness applied to the formula. Nothing worked.

When James was 23 months we had an occupational therapy appointment. I loved his OT. She was efficient, loud, and loved the kids she worked with. About halfway through our appointment she looked up and asked me, "When does James get his G-tube?" I was so stunned I just looked at her. I had been asking feeding therapies for a feeding tube for almost a year, with no success. With no reply from me she continued, "You are getting one right? Mom, he needs this." And I started to cry. Then I went on to thank her, and told her the process we had been through so far, and that I couldn't convince them that he needed this.

She scheduled a feeding clinic for us that very afternoon, with herself included. She fought for me when I was at the end of what I could do. At the end of this appointment she had a referral done up for us to receive and ng placement as soon as possible, and the referral done for the actual G-tube placement. Wow. I walked out feeling a huge weight taken off my shoulders.

I had just arrived back at my moms, about a fifteen minute drive through the city, when my cell phone rang. It was our OT. She had called the hospital, and we were to go to Royal University Hospital the next morning to have our ng placed.

If you've ever seen a child have an ng placed, you know how awful it is. An ng is a small tube placed up the nose and down the throat into the stomach, a safe way to place liquid into the stomach. No aspiration! One nurse and one student nurse were going to do the original placement, then pull it, and I had to learn before we could go home in case he ever pulled it out at home. After watching the student nurse freak out and repeatedly freeze while that tube was up his nose I kicked her outta the room. Just imagine, a child crying so hard he was puking up phlegm (I didn't feed him before coming in!), fighting with all his strength to get off the bed, me and the nurse holding him down, and nursing student crying over him pushing that tube in and out and then freezing. I'm all for teaching, but my child wasn't going to be the guinea pig! With her out of the way, I straddled James, holding his head with one hand and arm, my other arm holding his arms, and my body holding his tiny body down. And the nurse waiting for him to breathe in, and in the tube went. Done! Oh crap. My turn. Shit.

  I mustered all my strength and courage, rambled a frantic prayer, pulled that ng out, waited for that big inhale, and put that ng tube in perfectly! And then proceeded to do so about eight times every day! He was a pro at pulling that tube out every single time I wasn't watching him, no matter how well I had taped it to his face, and I was a pro at pinning him down by myself, waiting for that deep inhale, and jamming it back in! After about a week of this, I realized I would save myself a lot of work, and his face a lot of tape, if I simply placed the ng for feeding times, and then took it out myself in between! Four weeks later, once we knew the tube feeding was a very effective solution to his feeding problems, we returned to Royal University Hospital in Saskatoon and did the G-tube surgery.

  The surgery went well, taking less than an hour. He came out of anesthetic horridly, as was expected. The nurses called me into recovery as soon as he came in, knowing his wake up was going to be rough, and they were going to need me there. I knew when to turn his tiny jerking body on its side when he began choking, all while his jaw was locked and he was screaming. The rest of the time I simply stroked his hair and tried to console him, until his body slowly started to loosen up.

I cried when I saw his tiny bleeding belly with a horrific hole in it afterwards. What had I done? After two sleeps in the hospital, and enough confrontations with the nursing staff to last me a lifetime, I may have possibly went slightly ballistic on the nurse who insisted on feeding James pure formula, at a much higher rate than was realistic after surgery, and then telling me that we would be here for weeks if he didn't stop throwing up his feeds! I'm not a very tolerant momma when someone doesn't follow my instructions when it comes to his basic care. Let's just say when doctor rounds were done, I gave them the run down on being sick of being ignored, explained that I was more than capable of caring for my child at home, and threw in a few less than child appropriate words and several tears. He signed our discharge papers right there! I waited for the dietician to come up so I could ask a few questions about daily calories and oral foods, and we were on our way!

While this was a long fight to accomplish, I learnt a lot about myself going through this. James was mine, and he was a gift. And my judgement for him was good. I prayed for this child every day. Every time I had to do something for him or to him. Every time there was a decision to be made, an appointment to go to. I could trust myself to listen to the answers to my prayers, without always seeking outside direction.

The site around the G-tube healed very well. Granulation tissue became an issue, and steroid creams didn't help. My doctor prescribed silver nitrate to burn the granulation tissue, and told me how to protect the skin around it to keep the burn from travelling. Once I knew how to do this well, granulation tissue was no longer an issue and we never had any more problems. And I could burn off any warts that Julia go on her feet without having to see a Dr!

James' appointments were becoming exhausting. We all dreaded them. This was when I made a decision that has guided how I have raised James. I stepped back from my appointments. No more therapy appointments every week. We did our paediatrician, eyes, ears, orthopaedic surgeon, neurology, and so on, every six months or every year, or as needed. Our feeding clinics, occupational therapy, physical therapy, speech language therapy, G-tube clinics, were all done every three to six months now, and I carried out what I felt needed to be done daily at home. The nurses at Royal University Hospital showed me how to change the g-tube, and we now only go back if we have concerns.

As for feeding, occupational therapy, physical therapy, and speech language, my view is this. It came down to what kind of life I wanted for James. Did I want a life so crammed full of appointments, and hours upon hours of stretches and exercises every day? Or did I want to take the one thing that gave James pure joy, being with people, and fill his little heart so full with love and time and laughter, that his life couldn't possibly feel any more joyful? I chose the latter. And I have done so with much judgement from others. However, this continues to be my stance.

This is by no means saying that I do not take what these therapists have to say to heart! It simply means that I take in everything they have to say, and I step back and look at my son, and our family, and I pick and choose. Some of their suggestions I take and make our own, and run with them, taking them farther than they would have imagined! And some of them, I simply set aside. I know my child, and I trust that now.

At the time that this decision was made, we were still so unsure how long we would have James with our family. We made a decision to place quality in front of quantity. And today, James is seven years old, and so strong and healthy! And our decision remains the very same. Our little boy loves people, so our focus is on communication. How can we help him to communicate? How can he best interact with the world and people around him? And we fit in those necessary stretches around diaper changing and clothing changes. He gets time in his AFO's and standing frame daily. He goes to gymnastics and bowling and swimming. And he is happy. So happy. Our therapists are happy with where he is at, and how we have chosen to do things for him.

{2015} Years later, and this is still the best decision I have ever made. Quality over quantity. James has thrived beyond our craziest dreams. And all regular appointments have now been cancelled. His specialists now include: family doctor, pediatrician, occupational therapist, two physiotherapists, speech language and communication therapists, feeding and nutrition, orthotics, and orthopaedic surgeon. One physiotherapist comes into his classroom and sets up a program, which is carried out daily with him. She informs me when she is going in and lets me direct anything I would like to see them working on, and we talk regularly on the phone. He sees his pediatrician and orthopaedic surgeon annually. Other than that, every appointment is now parent directed. I call when I need them, and we either come to an agreement about something over the phone, or an appointment is scheduled. I have a great relationship with all of his doctors and therapists.

I turned 7!
{October 22, 2014}

Today James turned seven! My heart was so incredibly full. I cried often today, but really, what else is new?! It started with holding him before placing him in his chair for his morning feed. I danced with him and sang happy birthday, and he just melted into me and giggled! Precious.

We got to school that morning, and keep in mind that we are new to the city we are living in, and James has only been attending here for a little more than a month. Every single teacher's aide and teacher in the room stopped what they were doing and yelled "happy birthday James" as we came around the corner! He was delighted! Those little legs were tensed up and straightened in front of him, his arms pulled up to his chest, and he squealed! His teacher was at the counter pouring cupcake batter into molds for a birthday party that afternoon for James.

He came home on the bus, with a backpack full of gifts, and cards, and his notebook said that today he played in the ball pit all morning, and had a birthday party, complete with a bouncy castle and cupcakes that afternoon! Yes, pureed cupcakes ☺ He was so happy and excited! Grandparents and siblings and my best friend all called to talk to him on the phone, and he was so happy to hear them sing happy birthday to him!

I had his feeding chair all decked out with helium balloons and a gift bag beside the chair for him, thinking we would do presents with cake! Nope! As soon as he was hooked up for his supper feeding, he was yelling at me for that gift bag! Up until now he really hasn't understood presents at all. So, I didn't deny him, it's his birthday after all. So I picked up the bag, and handed him the stuffed bear on top. But he didn't take it from me – he just nodded NO very clearly! What?? Why didn't he want the bear? So I put it on the table, and he cleared shook his head NO again!! Now I was confused! So, I put the bear back in the back, and he smiled and yelled at me!! I put the whole gift bag on his tray, lying it down, so he could see inside.

And what James did next was our birthday miracle. That boy, who previously had no clue what presents were, reached into that bag, and slowly, very slowly, pulled out every single thing, right to the bottom of the bag. He opened his own present! And he knew it was for him!!! What?! I have waited seven years for this day!!

Then he yelled at me to hand him the cards he had received at school so he could show me! What?! This boy knew it was his birthday! It was his seventh birthday, and for the first time, he knew. The tears flowed today.

The day ended with birthday cake. A chocolate cream cheese pie with soft crust, because who wants to eat pureed cake for your own birthday?! He loved it! Then a huge pillow couch made by his sister, where they laid together, watching full house and playing with the helium balloons that she had tied to each of their wrists.

My heart was so full today! We didn't go out and do anything big – he was far too tired after his day at school. But this little miracle knew, he KNEW it was his birthday. AND he knew those presents were for HIM. AND he opened them himself. HUGE.

My miracle fell asleep peacefully on the couch tonight. After a day where I knew he felt loved all day. Pretty much a dream come true.

Now that James is seven, I feel like my world is again changing. My struggles are now centering around the long run. When he turns eight will I be able to lift him from the couch to his bed? When he is eight, where will I change his diaper when we go out? When he is eight, will he still be cute? Will his cuteness still win over the outsiders, making him feel like he somewhat belongs?

The most prevalent struggle? Will James learn to communicate? He is seven, and still so very trapped in his very own world. Will he learn to break out? Am I doing enough to help him break out? How can I help him to be the most successful he can be in life? Is he feeling valued and like his life has worth?

There is always that background fear that some cold or flu strain will invade his skinny little body, and be too much for him to overcome. Someday I will lay my sweet boy to rest. However, he has become so much stronger than I ever thought possible. And now my mind wanders more towards.... what if.... just what if.... this skinny little trapped determined boy.... outlives me. Or my capabilities. What if the day comes when that sweet boy rolls over my grave in his wheelchair. Heaven forbid. What if he rolls over my husband's grave too. While this is a normal aspect of most people's lives, I pray every day, that I will outlive James, by just one day. I only want to know that grief for a single day, before that sweet boy RUNS into my arms in heaven. On that day I will not lift him from his wheelchair. Nope. My boy will RUN to me. I will hear him say the word "mom". I might hear the words "I love you". I cannot even imagine what that will feel like!

James requires every aspect of care provided for him. Hygiene, feeding, communication, all mobility. He is completely vulnerable, especially because he isn't able to communicate verbally the way I would. If I am gone, is someone going to watch out for my boy? Will he be loved in every aspect of his daily care, or will he become a chore? A paycheck. Something in the way of someone's coffee break at work. Who will ensure that he isn't being physically or sexually or emotionally abused. Will someone take the time to hug him when he is having a stressful day? Will anyone take the time to even know he is having a stressful day?

Will anyone make sure that his diaper is dry late at night so that he doesn't lie in that all night? Will someone watch his spine, to make sure those bruises aren't starting to breakdown? Will anyone cut his toe nails so he doesn't split them while kicking, causing infection? Will anyone clean those extra waxy ears, or make sure his nose is clear, so that he is socially presentable?

Will anyone bother to help him with the bean bag toss at the fair? Or sweet talk the ride operator into waiting while they transfer James into the ride from his wheelchair and get positioned beside him, holding him safely, so he can feel the wind in his hair and giggle like the rest of the people at the amusement park?

Will his diaper be changed with dignity? Will the adequate time be taken to make sure his skin is dry with cream applied before the clean diaper is put on? Or will skin breakdown and rashes and infection be inevitable?

Will anyone make him a soft cheesecake for his birthday when I am not there? Will they fill balloons with helium and attach long ribbons so he can lie on the floor and play with them?

All of this weighs on my heart. Every. Single. Day.

This may sound like a lot of worry, which is useless. And not only is it useless, undealt with, I believe it becomes a sin. I am supposed to be giving my worries over to God, who will carry the burdens for me! However, I do not consider this simply worry. It is my reality. As James becomes older I find myself worrying about the future more, usually unconsciously. I have worked exceedingly hard over the last few years to overcome worry. Living everyday worrying about the future is a terrible way to live. I have managed to come out of that stage of my life. However, when you are raising a child who is totally dependent upon you for survival, the reality of your future cannot be avoided. The reality that he will never live an independent life. This is all the reality of my world, and I strive to turn my worry into preparation, a soft heart, and thankfulness every day.

I have worked a few jobs in the last few years that would allow me a glimpse into his future if there came a time when I was no longer physically able to care for his needs, or had passed away. I spent some time working in an institution for adults with physical and mental disabilities, and in a day program for adults with moderate to severe mental and physical disabilities. There were situations that were so encouraging, and situations that broke my heart and instilled fear. I have seen staff who adopt these people as their own family. They take the time to listen to them, they ensure their personal care is done with dignity and respect. They interact with them on their level, and look for ways to go above and beyond what is required for the job to better their quality of life.

But I have also seen the opposite. They are often dressed sloppily because those are the fastest clothes to get onto their frail or rigid bodies. Their diapers are only changed once if it is absolutely necessary, or they have leaked through to their clothing, causing skin breakdown. The changing can be done in such a hurry that they are not properly cleaned, causing them to stink. Feeding is rushed and so far from enjoyable, because someone else wants a few extra minutes of coffee break. But none of this is considered abuse. It's working within the deadlines and staffing limitations, and it is everywhere.

Just before James' fifth birthday I became very ill. It started with a pain that radiated throughout my entire body, for days. A few days in, my fever spiked. I ran a high fever for weeks. After about a week of fevers, I was bound to the couch. The pain in my body was unbearable. I was completely dehydrated. I couldn't keep any food or drink down and I was too weak to drink or eat anymore. There was an entire week where I barely moved from the couch, except for four trips to the emergency room. My husband and my best friend each took me to the hospital twice. My parents came up twice to help out around home. John missed days of work. My best friend came over to help around the house.

I could see life happening around me, but I was suddenly unable to interact with it. I could hear things happening, but I couldn't respond. I couldn't talk. I couldn't process. I could barely move. I had no strength and no ability to communicate back to anyone. I remember very little from that week, only snap shots of moments.

Visit after visit to the emergency room turned up no answers. Each time they would do blood work, xrays, and cat scans. Then they would rehydrate me through iv, give me very strong pain medication through the iv, and send me home. They knew I would be back, so they began leaving my iv port in to prevent having to reinsert it the next time I was back. After being rehydrated and relaxed with medication I was able to walk, with assistance, back to the van to ride home. Where I would return to the couch.

On my second last visit, the neurologist was called. He had looked at all my bloodwork and scans, and was fairly certain that I had viral encephalitis. In which case, there was no treatment further than what we were already doing. He asked me to return to the emergency room the next day to meet with him.

The next day I came back, and he did a full assessment with me. He diagnosed it as viral encephalitis, and said the important thing was that the fever leaves, as that is where the damage happens. The fever at this point was already much lower, and I felt my fog slightly lifting. I went home with instructions to return if I needed liquids, pain medication, or if my high fever returned and stayed longer than a day.

The high fevers subsided, but it took two more weeks before I was off of the couch. This for me was far scarier than the cancer ever was. I didn't know what it was for so long, and once we did know, we knew that it was serious, and could turn at any point. Lying on the couch, unable to respond to your surroundings, worrying about the future of your dependent son, is something that I wish on no one. It hurt my heart so deeply and I couldn't even share my fears. My best friend would come to visit me, but the only thing I remember is her taking my hand. I only remember having a hand to hold, when my mind was so loud and so afraid, but I couldn't speak any words. I wasn't afraid for me. I was afraid for James. For everything that I have said.

There is something surreal about being responsible for another life. And really every mother is. However, once the child is one, their independence is always increasing. We need to do less and less for their basic survival needs. They learn to take care of themselves. They learn how to seek help. They learn how to stand up for themselves, protect themselves. My baby cannot do any of that. I know instinctively like no one else when something is not right in his world. The thought of him not having that is the heaviest thing I have ever felt.

But for now, my miracle fell asleep peacefully on the couch. After a day where I knew he felt loved all day. Pretty much a dream come true.

And I will tuck him in snuggly under his favorite blankets. And kiss him a few extra times. And be thankful that he turned 7 today.

What Did You Just Say?

My whole world changed when I had James, and it took me a long time to let myself step into what was healthy for us, and step away from what was unhealthy for us. To trust myself enough to be able to do that; and for my heart to be peaceful with whatever that looked like. Sometimes people are intentional with their reactions to us, and sometimes they aren't; sometimes nothing has changed other than how I may feel in that environment; and I am now able to easily distinguish between the two.

When James was a baby I was attending a once weekly moms and tots group. Moms and their young children would gather together on Thursday mornings, together with more mature moms, for a time to support and encourage each other and learn together. The children would be in a room next to us playing with college students, and the babies would stay and roll around the centre of the circle or be passed around for others to hold. At this time, we did not have a diagnosis for James, we simply knew that things were not right. We knew about the cCMV, but nothing further. I went every week, so very exhausted, worried, stressed, and alone. Babies were very accepted and loved within this group, except James. I would hold James most of the time; no one would ever ask to hold him. Sometimes I would lie him down because I was so exhausted, and people would avoid making eye contact with him, like he had a disease that they would catch. I can name two, maybe three people, in that large group, who acknowledged James.

I continued to show up, week after week. Week after week I opened my heart, and week after week I went home broken and cried. I still believed things would change and I continued to go, until it felt as though I was being targeted. At the end of each week, we would spend time in prayer for one another. And one week, one girl shared, as she looked me in the eye, that she was just so thankful for all our healthy babies, and she gave thanks for that in prayer. And this happened again the next week.

I am a fairly strong girl, but I could not hold my tears in. Before that prayer even started, my eyes were so full. My heart was so broken. And so I made the decision that continuing to open my heart week after week, only to feel James and myself being rejected, was no longer in our best interest.

After being absent for a few weeks, I received a phone call from someone in the group, inquiring as to why I had stopped coming. I told her only a little about how James was being treated so differently and that it was too hard on my heart to watch week after week. I felt a peace about being honest, and waited for an encouraging response. But an encouraging response was not what I received at all. What was said to me still rings in my ears. "Dawn, you clearly have a jealousy issue. And if you cannot be a part of a group like this without being so openly jealous of all the healthy children, then maybe this isn't the group for you until you have worked on this sin in your life."

Really? Really??? I had never shown anything but love for every other mother's children there. And that is all I would ever show. I explained that I was sorry she felt this way, said that I had nothing but love for those children, and gracefully said that I wouldn't be coming back to the group. This person remained in the same community as we did for the next seven years, and never made mention of this again. Never invited me back. Never apologized for such a hurtful accusation.

These situations become something that is dealt with far more than I have ever or will ever talk about. Even writing about such specific situations makes me slightly uncomfortable. Whether they realized what their comments meant or not I will never really know, but they broke pieces of my heart that never fully come back. And so many moms have been through this heart break. Just knowing that you are not alone makes the walk just a little bit easier.

Another day that I remember so clearly was in the midst of the unknown, when James was so tiny, we had no clear answers, and the days and nights were indistinguishable and so hard. In talking with a friend on a Sunday morning, she asked how I was doing. I opened my heart and was honest about my hurt and fatigue, and her reply broke me. She said, "well, we all have our things to deal with in life." I had just been so honest about really hard, personal things, and she was my friend, not an acquaintance. Her response was so impersonal, so cold. At the time, it felt hurtful, spiteful. While I still don't think the response was right, I also no longer believe that she meant to hurt me. Maybe the realness of my response was too much? Maybe there was something happening in her life that I had no idea of, and she didn't feel like she could impose on me at that time? Maybe she had no idea how to respond to the depth of heart ache that I had just shared with her? Whatever the reason, whether it was right or it was wrong, I know that it wasn't fueled by negativity.

Not always have I handled negative reactions to my life well. One day I was shopping in Safeway with James when he was about three. James was born a puker. Right from day one that boy could projectile vomit like no one you've ever seen before. Everyone who has ever seen him puke is amazed by the volume and force. He does not vomit because he is sick; he vomits because he was born with congenital cytomegalovirus (cCMV), and one of the results of that virus is that he has a hard time digesting food, and he vomits regularly. Regularly as in ALL THE TIME. When he was younger, he did it at least three times a day. So, on this day, he and I were in Safeway quickly picking up a few things. We hadn't slept in weeks. I was a walking zombie. He had been crying so much. I was an emotional wreck.

We were walking down the card aisle, looking for a mother's day card. And James started to choke. And wretch. Oh no – please God – don't let this happen in the grocery store. Please. More choking. Now I'm fumbling to get a blanket and spread it out fast enough to create a cape from his neck out, to catch the projective storm that was about to erupt. I'm also on the verge of tears. There's a lady close to us also looking at cards, who looks disgusted, and moves farther away from us.

James puked. Oh my goodness he puked! I had to get a second blanket to catch a second wave of it!! It was so much that it went right through the blankets! I just had to crumple them up and stuff them under the stroller. Then this lady walked past us – pressing up against the other side of the aisle as to not get too close to us, and she says under the breath, but most definitely wanting me to hear, "the nerve, bringing a sick child out to where people buy their food." That was my breaking point. I wasn't thinking clearly from the lack of sleep. I snapped. I replied loudly enough and stern enough for her to know I was angry, with enough tears for her to probably consider reporting me to the mental hospital, but quiet enough to remain discreet amidst all the other shoppers. I quickly and directly told her that my baby was born with severe brain damage, and that he wasn't sick, but rather that this was our life. And I hadn't slept in years because I am up 24/7 caring for his every need. Well, that poor lady just stood there, mouth open, no words, and I turned and walked away. I probably stormed away quite childishly actually. And then I stopped in the next aisle to cry again.

Now I know that it would have been much more productive for me to simply explain to her kindly our situation, and likely she would have apologized, and thought twice before judging the next scene without any information on those people's lives. However, sometimes when you've had no sleep and life feels out of control, stupidity gets met with stupidity, and for just a moment, you feel better!

I took my daughter to swimming lessons one day. Once I had her in her bathing suit I sent her out to wait for her teacher, and I wheeled James out to the pool deck in his wheelchair and found a place to sit and watch. Beside us were another young mom and her daughter, maybe four years old, also watching the swim lessons. I sat down, got out James' feeding bag, and hooked him up to his feeding pump. Now this is fairly discreet. His feeding tube is under his shirt, and there is simply a line that leads to a bag (the same as an iv bag), and a fairly quiet pump. I input the pump settings, hit run, and no big deal – he is now eating. All you can see is a small line running from the feeding bag to under his shirt. The mom beside us watched this, wide eyed, and then shot me the dirtiest of looks, picked up her daughter, and went and sat all the way across the pool from us!

Can you say ignorant? But whatever, I had no reaction this time. Oh I was disgusted! But I didn't show it. And if I was honest, it did hurt my heart. It hurt my heart because some people are so closed minded to anyone who is different. And they teach those around them to be the same way. James' tube isn't scary! Often Julia's friends come over and see James hooked up to his pump. When they look at it, I ask if they would like to see his feeding tube and know more, and they always say yes! So I take the opportunity to show them his actual mic-key button, and explain how the food goes directly into his tummy, and why it has to happen that way. When Julia was younger I would also let her friends' parents know that I had shown them. Once a child has seen it all, it isn't scary to them at all! They usually think it is quite cool! And they just seem to understand that this is what he needs, and they never think twice about it again when they see me feed him.

The more people we can educate with love, the more their hearts are going to change towards people that are different from them. People are often scared of James because of the amount that he drools. And really, that's fair if you have never been around someone like that before. He drools like a fountain! And as much as I try to keep up and keep his hands, face, bib, clothes, and general surroundings dry, he's just so darn good at replicating old faithful! I try to keep extra dry bibs with me at all times, and blankets for wiping it from his face, and for him to hold. The cleaner I can keep him, the less afraid of him people seem to be.

Every once in a while I meet someone who, just in general conversation, reaches over and either with James' bib or blanket, wipes his chin for him. This blows me away. Want to speak my love language? That simple act speaks my love language louder than anything else. Not being afraid of his ridiculously adorable little face, and doing something to make him more comfortable, melts me. I may hug you. I've learned to restrain as that freaks people out! But if you see me eyeing you up for a hug, you just might be my very next victim.

There's also the other extreme; the people who are so comfortable with your child that they are crossing boundaries. Some people think that because he cannot verbalize a no, that his head shaking no response means less than a person who has said a firm no. If you ask him to hold his hand or give you a high five, and he reaches out, then by all means, please do. However, if you ask to give him a high five, and he vigorously shakes his head no, that does not mean he's inviting you to kiss him on the forehead! How would you like it if some stranger came up to you, and like in a bad dream you were unable to verbally respond to them, or run away like you wanted to, so they just grabbed your face with their hands and gave you a big smooch? My child has every right to say no to that, just like any other child. Just because he is in a wheelchair and adorable doesn't mean he wants your hands on him.

So far I have never freaked out on anyone for this, but please don't try to be the first person that I do lose it on. So far I have been able to ward people off by simply putting my arm between them and James and telling James to wave goodbye, while I push him away.

Lego and Nerf Guns..... Maybe?
{ November 7, 2014}

    Would James play lego? Would he chase his sister through the house, laughing mischievously, shooting her relentlessly with the biggest nerf gun he could find? What would his voice sound like if words and sentenced flowed from his mouth?

    I wonder all these things as I listen to the sound of lego being dumped on our floor, and nerf guns being shot in every direction. Not usual sounds in my basement! But today my daughter has a young boy from her class over to play.

At first I thought to myself, "boys are so loud! And exhausting! I should hug all moms that have boys!" Then my heart just sort of stopped. I have a boy.

    I have a boy. But I don't hear these things. And my heart broke. What I wouldn't give to hear these things everyday. Accepting this new life has been such a process. Such a grieving process. And I do not believe that it will ever be over, as long as James is with us.

    When James was born, we grieved the fact the he might become deaf and blind. Although after all those tests in the NICU, we were so relieved that was all we would be dealing with. The grieving was very minor... it really hardly phased us.

The grieving when the neonatologist, at 3 months of age, told us that James may not live, and if he did his quality of life would be so very low, was much more intense. Life sucking, heart stabbing, strength searing real. I cried so many tears, felt so hollow . Then the pieces started to fit together. We had some answers to the things that James was and wasn't able to do at this point. I had proof that I wasn't losing my mind. When people had questions, I had some answers. They were pretty vague answers, but they gave validation to my fears and tears and exhaustion and confusion.

Grief has different waves, and those waves are different in every situation. Different sizes, heights and depths, severity, and length. Acceptance is generally the last stage of grief. However, this time acceptance came around incredibly fast, there was almost no confusion or anger or questions following the initial news. My heart accepted what had been told to us graciously. I think my heart already knew. A mom's heart isn't usually too far off.

When James was diagnosed with spastic quadriplegia cerebral palsy, it felt a little bit harder. I felt like I now really had to accept what was happening, and my grieving really happened in this stage.

James and I, and my mom, attended a clinic at the Kinsmen Children's Centre in Saskatoon where we saw a physiotherapist, occupational therapist, and our pediatrician. Our pediatrician was the last appointment. In this appointment, she mentioned the cerebral palsy a few times as she spoke, but I wasn't really connecting the dots. At the end of the appointment she asked me if I had any questions. I was sitting on a child's orange vinyl and metal chair beside the hospital bed that James was lying on, and it took me a minute to speak. I remember very clearly asking, "So, are you officially giving him the diagnosis of cerebral palsy?" She looked gently into my eyes and replied "yes". She wrote the kind of cerebral palsy on a paper for me, and that is actually all I remember. At some point I would have gone back to my mom's to drop her off, and probably brought James inside to stretch before I made the 2.5 hour drive home.

Of that drive, I remember very little of the road. I remember my heart breaking. Feeling so alone and isolated and scared. I remember crying so hard that I was sobbing out loud, and I could barely see the road through my tears. I felt like a house had been dropped on my chest, I could barely breathe. At one point I remember looking up and seeing a construction worker, shaking his fist and yelling furiously at me. I had just driven through a construction zone with a speed of 60 km/h, right beside workers, at a speed of at least 120 km/h. But that didn't even fully register with me. I should not have been driving that evening alone, just James and I.

I do not process things fully until I have had time alone. So while I knew that this diagnosis was hitting me, I didn't know until we were driving that it was crushing me.

The next year was so hard. When I think back, I only remember snap shots from that whole year. Significant moments that stand out in my mind. Everything else is a huge emotional blur. My heart was right, things were not okay with my baby, and now that everyone was agreeing with me, it felt so final.

I grieved. I grieved hard, and long, and it was ugly. And for the most part, I did it alone. Not only did most people not know how to enter into that with me, I didn't know how to let anyone truly enter into that with me. Everything I had ever hoped for my son felt like it came crashing down and I had to let it all go. And I had to do that, while enduring and surviving the constant crying and screaming, the constant pneumonia, puke everywhere every single day, little to no sleep, almost no friends, and a three year old daughter full of spunk and attitude that required endless energy.

I fell to the floor crying, begging, pleading with God more times than I can count. I tried to barter my way out of this mess. God, if you do this, if you heal my boy, or heaven forbid, sometimes that deal included, if you take this boy home and release him from his constant pain, I will do anything.

I grieved when James got his g-tube, but as I saw his quality of life improve so drastically, that it went away quite fast. Even though I fought so hard to have this tube placement, there was a small part of me that grieved it, because enteral feeding is considered a form of life support. It was a reality that I knew we needed, but felt restricting.

I feel grief with every birthday, both his and mine, and every holiday. I know this is irrational and should not happen, but it does every single time, and I have to believe that I am not alone in this. I believe many moms in similar situations must feel the very same way, I've just never been able to have that conversation.

I feel it on my birthday because my life has changed so much from what I always, and still do, dream for myself. I am a creative person at heart, but I feel too exhausted most of the time to do much with it. I will have a month of great sleeping patterns with James and I will start feeling like I'm getting my feet back under me, and then, at 7.5 years old, he won't sleep again for weeks on end. And all my dreams and creative plans are forgotten all over again. I feel it on my birthday because I have changed so much, out of necessity.

I feel it on his birthday too, which of course I do not talk about, because I am also so thankful for the milestone! I am so thankful for each year, and I would feel like the most terrible parent ever to express anything but that on his birthday. It is also a reminder of everything that he cannot do. Of the birthday parties he has never gone to. Of everything that we cannot do with him. Of everything that I long so deeply to give him, but will never be able to. It reminds me of the toy aisle that I should be shopping in for him, but brings me to the toy aisle that is appropriate for his abilities. With each birthday I am still pureeing food, changing diapers, and lifting his boney long body into a wheelchair.

I feel it on every single holiday. New Years, Easter, Thanksgiving, Christmas. While most people are looking forward to the down time, the sleeping in, and family time, church services, family traditions, time with friends, I am seeing all of the work. I am exhausted at the end of a normal day, but add on top of that travelling to see family, bringing along everything needed. The sleep that I don't get, while everyone else does. The traditions and outings that aren't made to easily include James, but finding ways to include him. The joy in people everywhere, and somehow I have this grief. I long to be hugged, just a little longer than usual, and to just simply be allowed to not be ok for a minute. To not have it all together for a moment. To admit the grief. But I still haven't learnt how to do that.

I grieve on the first day of school each year. I have always been so thankful for the programs that have been in place for James, and I continue to choose these over inclusion. But wheeling his chair into the school that first morning each September feels a little bit like a knife to my chest. I lose my breath for a moment. My eyes usually glaze over more than once. All the running and screaming and hugging and chatter amongst friends, reminds me that James does not have that. He has teachers and aides that are amazing and do so much to welcome him, but it does not replace a child running up to your child, hugging them, taking their hand and running away. Seeing that your child has a place and belongs and has a friend that is there with them and for them; James never has that. And my heart breaks every single time.

I grieve momentarily every day. James is 7.5 years old, and loves to sit in his Rifton Activity chair, in our large living room window, and watch the traffic, and people walking, and our neighbors. And every day I smile and feel so much joy that he feels joy when he is there. And every day I walk by and struggle to breath, because I want more for him.

    I grieve when we have a day of back to back appointments. Partly because all of the children there are in similar situations as James, and you realize that you are forever a part of this community. And this community is amazing! You just never plan to be a part of it. It is also because there are always things they feel that I should be doing better, doing more, doing less. More things I should be trying, things I am doing that they think aren't beneficial for him. Sometimes it is hard to weigh it all, and feel confident in the decisions you have made. And so there is a form of grieving there, and you weigh the options, and chose the best one for your child, you and your family.

    I write this because I would assume that there are so many parents out there like me, who feel this weird grief that seems to surface on holidays. That makes them want to hide until it is all over. That screams out for a place to let go, to cry, to grieve, not alone, but having no idea how to ask for that. My hope is that you will read this, and feel less alone.

Faith

Blog Entry {March 16, 2011} Break my heart until....I'm still

  Sometimes I feel so inadequate because of the hurt that I feel each day. I have recently come to a place where this is ok. Romans 5: 3,4 "Not only so, but we also rejoice in our sufferings, because we know that suffering produces perseverance; perseverance, character and character, hope."
  Just yesterday, while John was changing James, he noticed several sores on his back and called me over. Heart breaking. He is so thin that he has sores on each of his vertebrae on his back. I love this little boy more than words can express. And my heart shatters each and every day for his tiny body. My heart shatters when we eat, and he opens his mouth as we do. My heart shatters when his sister runs by with a friend, and he cries, wanting so badly to play with them. My heart shatters when his body jerks him awake from sleep, terrifying him. My heart shatters when we talk about the future surgeries he will need. These hurts are not

going to stop. I struggled with knowing how to go on in the midst of the daily hurt for so long.

This somewhat sums it up.... "Break my heart until.... I'm still" In the midst of such deep hurt, I am still. I'm rarely still. But when that hurt comes into my heart, everything else stops momentarily. And in that stillness, my Savior meets me. He knows my hurt. If I love this little boy so much that my heart shatters daily, how much more does Jesus love my little boy? These moments of heart break give me the strength to keep going.

I write this today feeling a lot of different things. I turned 30 yesterday. (DEEP BREATH) I'm feeling old!! I'm feeling thankful for forgiveness and second chances, and friendships that God has restored to more than I ever knew they could be. I'm feeling thankful for a husband that has walked through some pretty dark valleys with me, and still seems to love me more every single day.

And I'm feeling really burdened. In the last 2 years, I haven't taken the time to really listen to my God. To follow where he wants me to be. This relationship has become very real and alive, and the things he is laying on my heart still aren't clear. But I'm open and willing, and excited!

Blog Entry {February 23, 2011} Always be kinder than you need to....

I read this somewhere a while ago..... "Always be kinder than you need to be to others. Everyone is going through something." This has really stuck with me. When I look around at the circles I interact with, it's so easy to just brush the surface. It's amazing how only taking a few moments out of your day to listen to someone's heart can really make a difference.

I've met a few people in the last week that have really impacted me. I met a beautiful young lady last week, who has been very hurt in life. She is not the first person you would gravitate towards in a crowd because she has withdrawn. I also met a new young mother who appears to have "everything" you could possibly want in life, but is just starting down the path of learning what difficulties her baby girl may face.

It's funny how in both circumstances, the tendency is to avoid the real. You can tell the first girl has real hurts, and it's easier not to go there. You can't tell that the second girl is going through anything, yet her heart is broken and she feels so lonely.

Jesus has commanded us to LOVE. Sometimes love is going for a half hour coffee with someone and just listening. Sometimes love is leaving your comfort zone, maybe not gravitating towards your usual group of friends, to get to know someone else just a little. I know I always go straight to where I am comfortable, to my group of friends. I've made it my goal to pray before going into settings like this (church, my husband's school, my children's schools), and to be more approachable. I'm not approachable if I beeline for where I'm comfortable. Not that there's anything wrong at all with spending the majority of your time with those you know and love. But I am feeling called to ask for God's grace, humble myself, and intentionally love those that may be slipping through the cracks, even if everything looks perfect on the outside.

As you go about your day today, remember when you interact with others "Always be kinder than you need to be to people. Everyone is going through something." Even that cashier that just took 10 minutes to ring you through. And the girl in your class you clings to you even though you do everything possible to avoid her. You never know how big of a difference a friendly smile can make to someone's day.

I am a Christian. And I have struggled in my walk. I believe that being a Christian means having a personal relationship with Jesus Christ, and walking in that relationship, through good times and hard times. My spiritual life has been far from perfect, but regardless it is who I am.

I know that I cannot walk this life alone. And no relationship on this side of heaven will ever be enough to sustain me. And yes, I believe in a heaven and a hell. I believe in a God who is just. Who is firm, yet loving. I believe that choosing to follow him involves hard decisions and sacrifices; I believe it involves keeping a soft heart amidst a world where hearts have hardened and closed off.

I believe that the biggest influence you will ever have in someone else's life is how you make them feel when you are in their presence. It isn't about what you say, what you have or what you gave them. If you made them feel loved, safe, special, or important, that will stick with them. They will remember the difference in your encounter.

I believe in sharing Jesus' love, for everyone, in my actions. If they want to hear my words they will ask. If they want my advice they will ask. But most often, a smile can speak a thousand words. A helping hand can change a life. Kindness can remind someone that they are not worthless; their life has value.

I am now 34, and I probably have more questions now about my own faith than I have ever had in my life. But with life experience, and knowledge, comes more questions. I don't have all the answers, and my views and opinions on some things have certainly changed from when I was much younger, but my heart belongs to Jesus Christ. And I pray that my daily encounters exhibit this.

My faith has sustained me through some incredibly dark times. I have cried out again and again for strength, for hope, for sleep, for peace. I don't know how I would have made it through the last seven years if I did not have my faith. Having someone to talk to, day or night, about the rawness in my heart, brings a peace far beyond understanding.

Planning the Unplannable

Unplannable. It is another one of those words that I have decided I am allowed to make up! How on earth do you write a will, when you know that in this will, you have to leave your children to someone. Generally we pick a parent, or a sibling, or a friend, who in the event that both parents pass away, will step up and raise your child or children. But how do you ask someone when you know this is a complete game changer? And how do you even pick someone? You need someone strong enough physically to do all that you do every day; someone you don't need to worry about physically hurting themselves while caring for your disabled child. You need to pick someone who can handle the financial aspect of raising a disabled child. Although we have arranged for good life insurance coverage, there needs to be strong money management skills to make that last in order to give James the care necessary.

Most of the time, when someone agrees to be the guardian, that means until the child reaches the age of 18. As long as James is still alive, this is a life long commitment. James' care will not cease to be necessary at the age of eighteen. The struggles will be ever increasing and demanding.

The list of people who know James and love him for who he is isn't very long, and knowing how to do this is still so hard. We want to pick someone who will fight for him. Someone who will know when the best thing for him is to go into a home, and who will spend the time and energy making sure to pick the very best placement for him, and to then stay involved in all decisions that affect his care, and stay active in his life as a loving parent. Someone who values their faith and values church life, and involves my children in that. Someone who values that relationship that James and Julia have, and will always keep them close.

We have spent so much time thinking about this topic, and trying to decide how to do it best. James is 7 and we still do not have one! We do now have a plan, and we desperately need to put it into writing. However, before we can put anything into writing, we need to have several conversations with people, which feels so hard to do. Which is why I still haven't tackled it.

We have decided to do a list of people, who have said yes, knowing that if the time ever comes, our executor will go through the list. As they do so, knowing that their life circumstances may have changed, or James' care needs may have changed, they have the right to pass. And we have to trust that one person on our list will be in the right position at the time to feel confident in taking on our children.

This is one of the things I have struggled the most with. I have changed my entire life to care for James, and I know I cannot ask someone else to do the same. But it is terrifying to think of him not having what he has now forever. So my plan is to live a terribly boring life, in a bubble, and live forever! Better yet, I am going to become a vampire and live forever! James' skin is often cold anyways, so he likely won't even notice the difference in my skin temperature! However, while I am looking for my vampire to bite me, maybe I should get writing that will. Sigh.

How Valuable is My Life?

People imply a lot of different things when it comes to the value of a person's life. We show the value we place on someone's life by how we treat them. When you place a doctor, and a disabled adult side by side, the way that they are treated by others shows the value they place on their lives. This is true in society as a whole, not just in the world of disabilities. Do we always treat the man pumping our gas as well as we treat the principal at our child's school?

The topic of euthanasia has been a hot topic over the last year. Most of the discussion focuses around elderly and terminally ill patients. But I can tell you, any mother raising a severely disabled child, or chronically ill child, has had this conversation, although often only with themselves. The things we may think from time to time are not popular, or sugar coated, so we keep them to ourselves. From time to time, someone will speak openly from their heart; unfortunately this is often met with harsh judgment and anger, but that's the only reaction that they see. They never hear from the many families that may read what they wrote from their heart, and simply feel less alone in their journey. We feel scared of our feelings, fears, and thoughts from time to time; but sometimes, knowing you are not alone in those fears is what gives you the courage to keep on going.

We are often given the option to abort, if through tests, we know something is "different" with our babies before they are born. We are offered a chance to simply not take the extra measures when illness hits, or put our children on permanent life support measures, such as feeding tubes or tracheotomies. We have to measure daily pain and suffering, against the terrible alternative, which is removing whatever life support they are living on, and watching immeasurable suffering while their bodies naturally shut down. We see families lose all hope, exhausted from the constant fight and struggle, and give in to the heart breaking reality of taking their child's life in a way that we cannot fathom. And we judge them, not having a clue what this family has endured, the fights they are constantly losing, the support that they have reached out for time and time again, and been denied. I am not supporting this decision; I am simply saying that we do not see inside their reality.

For me, I didn't know that there was any issue at all with James while I was pregnant, so the issue of terminating the pregnancy was a non issue.

When it comes to simply not taking the extra measures, and letting James go naturally, instead of always fighting, I chose against that. I was offered the option of foregoing the feeding tube, as things were going to get worse anyways. The thought that someone would offer this to me angered me, repulsed me, sickened me. I didn't give that a second to take seed in my mind, and very clearly chose to go ahead with a life support option, a g-tube, which I believed would change his quality of life.

Further into my journey, I have heard from so many people in situations similar to my own, and how they feel about their decisions years later looking back. Some moms are happy that they pressed on, took the risk, and have kept fighting. Some have seen their children flourish far beyond their dreams. Some have seen their children suffer far beyond what most can imagine. Some have seen their stabilize, but the daily fight is exhausting and life draining.

I remember one mom sharing how she wasn't sure if she made the brave decision to keep her child and constantly fight for her, or if she had just sacrificed the lives of everyone else in their house. She was now divorced. Her other children were angry and she didn't have the time to devote to them like they needed. Professionals were now telling her that for the health of her daughter, and of herself, it was time to let her daughter go and put her into a home. She had spent the first ten years of her daughter's life fighting against all odds for her, and in the end she was still going to lose her, and she had ruined every relationship in her life.

I've heard moms express how hard it is when the children grow up. The older they get, the less support is available. We start to run out of equipment options, funding options, respite options. There is no longer the treatments and equipment available to offer us a hope that things will improve. We become less capable of lifting their bodies into such equipment. We start to spend our energy daily on things like dressing, hygiene and feeding, not leaving a lot extra for all the work it takes to go on outings. At first non accessible venues do not stop us. We can wheel their small wheelchairs almost anywhere, change their diapers in our vehicles, and lift their small bodies where their wheelchairs cannot fit. We can scoop them out of their chairs and hold them almost anywhere.

As they get bigger we cannot do these things as often, if at all. We start to lose our freedom. I already feel isolated and lonely. I try not to think about when my freedom entirely goes away. When his freedom of inclusion goes away.

Nobody tells us these things at the beginning of our journeys. Nobody mentions that when puberty hits, their cuteness goes away. Now they look like that awkward teenager, and we have to increase our daily hygiene routines to the point where it's exhausting, but that acne and facial hair is still going to be enough to keep even more people away from our babies.

The outside support goes away. The understanding and helping hands go away. You are left in a world where someone else's existence is dependent upon you and you alone, and you really have nowhere to turn when it all becomes too much.

I struggle to write these things down for you to read, because I do not live my life dwelling on these things, or even talking about these things. There is too much silence in our communities though. We all struggle in life, often with ugly, scary things, but we refuse to talk about it. I know when someone else has given me a glimpse into their reality, I always feel less alone. And that is why I share these hard things. I don't write any of this as a judgment either way on anyone's decisions. I write this as a glimpse into where these decisions are coming from.

I may have never struggled with the issue of aborting my pregnancy, and I never struggled with the decision when my doctor did give me that chance when James was so young, but my mind has struggled along the way. Thank God I did not know how little support I would find when I was given such an option. Thank God my heart was filled with fight and determination and such hope. When they are young, the support can be endless. You can attend regular appointments for every specialty and every therapy, and there are countless outside organizations you can look to for help. People want to support you however they can, because no one can stand to see a child suffer. But nobody tells you that it all fades. People forget about you once they are a toddler and the needs get old. Once they hit five it is a struggle to access therapies and specialists in a timely fashion. The equipment options begin slimming, the accessible options for outings are smaller. Diapering becomes something you have to plan for when you are not at home.

Thank goodness I did not know about the emotional and physical struggles we would face. And thank God we did not know about the financial reality we were stepping into. If we have any savings at all, or a reliable sellable vehicle, that needs to be used before any outside funding can be accessed for equipment that is vital to your child's care. As soon as you are just above the poverty line, but still in that first, lowest tax bracket, you lose funding for enteral formula. James' food costs are equivalent to a few adults. Because he is a paraplegic, his incontinent supplies are covered. However we just had to fight against the limits they placed on him. They limited him to seven diapers a day. Seven diapers a day, for a child who is tube fed, would mean that his skin would constantly be wet, leading to skin breakdown. Not to mention odors that you just cannot get rid of once they are not cared for properly.

Living in Canada and having free health care, and free medications for James is a blessing that I do not take for granted. However, the financial toll is overwhelming as a whole. I have continually tried to hold down jobs that I love and that pay well, but James is often sick and misses 2-5 days of school a month lately, meaning that I rarely work.

We have not been in the position yet where we have had to cross the bridge of, do we pull his tube, knowing without that without nutrition he would die, or do we fight every way possible? I dread this day, and it creeps into my mind sometimes, because I have seen this happen. There is no legal way to end that suffering. Sometimes these children go WEEKS without nutrition, because their body rejects it. They starve to death so slowly. Their bodies have spent their entire lives fighting, overcoming the odds against them. They are trained to fight and survive when survival isn't thought to be an option. And we have no laws to protect these poor innocent bodies from themselves. A time that we all hope will be peaceful and full of love as we say goodbye to our babies, knowing they will soon be pain free, is often weeks upon weeks of sickening torture, as their bodies cling to life, while suffering immeasurably on the inside, unable to express it on the outside. It's funny how society thinks this is an okay way for my baby boy to die, yet there's nothing in place for a parent to make an educated decision to be able to give the child the peaceful love filled experience that they have fought so hard all their life for and deserve.

I had more than one night, when James was much smaller, where the idea of ending his suffering would not leave my mind. I remember lying in bed one night in his room, with his tiny, jerking, tight, body beside me, his lungs raging as they had been for hours, sending him into fits of choking. I would turn his body to the side and support him as best I could until he stopped choking, and then he would jerk again, starting the crying all over again. I was helpless. He was inconsolable. It had been years of this. What if I put this pillow over his face? Just until he was quiet. Loosened up. His torment would stop. He would run in heaven. And laugh. And nothing would ever hurt again. I would sleep. I could close my eyes and just sleep. I could wrap my arms around him, while he was still warm, and fall asleep holding my peaceful baby, and we could cope in the morning. I could cope in the morning. He would be free.

I've never said this to a soul. I almost threw up writing this. I will wretch every time that I read these words. But these words are truth. These are the thoughts that we keep to ourselves. And because we refuse to talk about them, others feel alone, and those thoughts win.

Blessings

We have both been blessed so many times because of the life we are living with James, and we have seen James bless others in ways that we would have missed without him. I tend to be a very empathetic, observant, deep feeler. I am often able to catch on to emotions from others that most people would not clue into. And I am often amazed at how James can do the same, and respond with a compassion and love far deeper than I have the capability of doing.

I went out for supper with the bestie, my sister and James one night in downtown Saskatoon. We were nicely enjoying our visiting, feeding James while waiting for our meals, when we heard someone yelling from across the restaurant "Oh you're in trouble now!" First I noticed that James' eyes were locked on this gentlemen – then my eyes moved to the man making the scene. I was feeling very uncomfortable. He went on to continue making inappropriate restaurant talk with James from about 15 feet away, and by now James was laughing. He wasn't terribly clean, looked worn, and slightly drunk. He came over and began talking to James, and James' reacted with smiles and laughter. You could see the joy it was bringing the man, to the point where there were tears in his eyes.

He came over several times during our meal, and each time he would begin to touch James' hands, and then move to touching his face, at which point I would cut it off as politely as possible. Over the course of the evening we learnt that his girlfriend just left him and he was feeling very hopeless. He found a non judgmental soul in James who would simply listen and bring a joy that words cannot describe. James blessed this man in a way that no one else there could that night. On our way out, the man hugged both James and I and we went our separate ways.

You will often see the elderly take James' hands in theirs and simply hold them. You can see the joy that James has brought to them in their gleaming eyes, and James seems to be just as happy. And no one has spoken a word! Often they will both end up laughing! It is surreal to see.

We have seen people go out of their way completely to bring a smile to James' face. Our neighbor's came over one day, and offered to take James for a ride in their little two seater convertible! So we buckled James' car seat into the passenger seat, and off they went! They came back to our house about four times, and each time James would point and yell, implying that he wanted to go again, and off they would go! And he would laugh! What an unexpected blessing!

Relationships

Relationships are hard and complex in life normally. But once you are thrown into raising a disabled and very sick child, they become ridiculous to maintain. And I failed here time and time again, and am so very thankful for those relationships that have made it through.

You will notice that as I have written this book, I have not often talked about how my husband and I dealt with things together. And there is a very simple answer for that; it is because we did not do a lot of this together.

When we began to see that James was going to have a much different life than we had planned, we also became aware that the divorce rate for couples raising a child with severe mental and physical disabilities, was over 80%. 80% divorce rate. I think that possibly knowing this rate helped us get through, even though we did not always get through well.

There have been some times where we clung to each other and got each other through. But there were so many more times where we did it alone. We had the same information, but we processed it all so differently, and at different times, and that became the normal.

James is now seven and we are starting to heal our relationship. We made it, neither of us left, although I'm sure there were more times than either of us will admit, that we almost walked away. Maybe ran away. We aren't doing better now because James is doing better. We are doing better now because we have both had time to work on who we were, on who we have become, because neither of us is the same person anymore. We are able to see what almost happened to our family, and we want so much better for our family.

People always say that your closest friends need to be in the same life situation as you. It is easiest when your children are small if they also have littles; they will understand better what your priorities are, your needs, hurts, and weird found joys. But the opposite ended up being true for me. I found a best friend who was single and five years younger than me. And we fit perfectly together. She is a talented actress, musician, singer, athlete, gorgeous, tall and thin. I am none of those things! Most people ran when my life got complicated and unsteady; she stayed. We found ways to make it work, and we complimented each other's lives.

Relationships become so very hard to maintain during some phases of raising a disabled or sick child. There were times that I had nothing left to contribute to our friendship, and she stepped up and did it all. She made the trips to see me, spent the money when we would get away for a few days, made the phone calls. And there have been times where I have totally got this all down, and she has struggled, and then I stepped up and did the work. I drove to her, paid for things, made the calls, sent the letters.

This relationship fell apart during this time also. When James was born she lived almost four hours away from me. Two years later, she moved to the same small town and we were only five minutes apart for the next five years! The first year and a half of that five years we spent quite estranged. Our communication stopped, feelings were hurt, walls went up, and yet we spent that time so close geographically, but so far apart relationally. I mention this only to encourage you, that even if you are seeing a friendship that you need so desperately deteriorate, give yourself enough grace and time to be able to pick yourself back up, and then start the often very slow process of repairing that relationship that you need forever.

Often times when I am struggling with James, with how I am handling the never ending work with him, I forget to think about how others are doing, or about how my words or actions are affecting them, or our relationship. Often, the things that have hurt me the most, were unintentional by those who hurt me.

Make sure you have one friend that you can simply cry with. Sometimes tears are healing. Simply letting yourself fall with someone allows you to see clearly again and move forward. I have found that I don't need lots of surface level friendships, I don't do those well at all. I need only a few deep, honest relationships. I need that precious gift of time spent together.

If you are reading this and you are raising a child with a severed disability, or a chronic illness, remember to take time to invest in a friendship. A friend who lets you be you, allows you time to rest, rejuvenate, laugh, cry, and sleep. I try to get away at least twice a year with my bestie. Once we go camping in a tent in the Rocky Mountains. We sleep in, spend our days hiking or biking, and cook all our meals over the fire. We talk for hours, walk and hike for hours. We sit around a fire until the park ranger drives around and says we need to put out the fire. Then we crawl into our tiny two person tent, stinking like smoke, and sleep until whenever we wake up. Or until I wake up at 3am having a panic attack about a bear ripping our tent open and eating me – and the bear would definitely eat me since she can run much faster than I can!

When I feel trapped by the 24/7 needs of my children, and my lack of work options because my husband's job takes him away from the home so much that

I can never work outside of school hours, and around all appointments, I start to see how awesome her life is! She is involved in too many sports to list, and can go out with friends at any moment, and I start to envy all that freedom she has to go after the things she wants! This is usually where she balances me out, sharing all the things she's struggling with, and what she all sees that I have. Having a best friend in a completely different life situation has been the most amazing gift, and has gotten us both through a lot of hard situations.

It's so easy to feel guilt over investing in a relationship outside of your family unit, especially when so much is demanded and needed from you within your family. But learning to do this has sustained me. It gives me the break I need to come back refreshed and ready to continue. It's so easy to lose sight of why you are doing everything that you do every day.

Blog Entry {February 16, 2011} It's not you......It's me

I am 29 years old, and I am just now really learning this. I've struggled in the last 3 years, watching relationship after relationship crumble around me. Good friends, acquaintances, family, and even my marriage. The stress of having a baby that you fully expected to be healthy, and finding out that he will have so many struggles in his life, consumed me.

But when relationships fail, what's the first thing we say? "You didn't...", "why did you....", "I needed you to......", "you always.....", and the list goes on and on.

My marriage crumbled a year after James was born. I very clearly remember one morning, I was up with James most of the night and on the chair in the living room with him. John had just gotten up and was getting ready for school, and Julia was playing. I was exhausted. We hadn't slept in the same bed for months. I was with James every single night - he was completely incapable of sleep. I spent my days doing hours of physiotherapy, bottle feeding him 7 times a day, most of which he threw back up. Trying to count every calorie that went into his tiny body and guess how many from each feed came back up. Going to endless doctors and specialists appointments, getting test after test done on him. Trying to find quality time to spend with my daughter, who was 3 at the time. Trying to have patience with her, and trying to make the days fun. John was a full time student and I worked evenings. That morning we both sat at the kitchen table, having the conversation that I will never forget. "Maybe we should separate for a while. Who will leave? Where should we go?"

Most of my friendships dissolved around the same time. I felt so abandoned by everyone that I thought would stay by my side through everything.

I started realizing that I wasn't the person I wanted to be anymore. I started to see that my heart was so closed. And I started praying that my heart would soften, that those walls would please please just start coming down.

John and I are the strongest today that we have ever been. And not because I changed him. I had to change my heart. And it has been a process. I have been consciously working on this for almost 2 years now, and finally feeling the results.

I still have broken relationships. But I am slowly picking up some of the pieces, and seeing the areas that I need to work on. It took me almost 2 years, but I am just now able to open my heart back up, and take a few chances. I'm not finding it incredibly easy. I probably seem much less emotionally stable now than ever before actually. I went to superstore the other night, and cried when I paid for my groceries! Today I stopped to pick up a few things there, and got the same cashier. She remembered me, and said "are you feeling any better today dearie?"

Embarrassing when you have a line up of people behind you!

It seems crazy to be learning such important life lessons still. My life would have been sooooooo much easier if I wasn't so stubborn, and could have learned this much younger. I may not be trying to piece together as many things as I am.

I am thankful for a God who forgives, and who allows us to forgive. I am thankful that with His strength and grace, I am learning to be humble and honest and vulnerable.

I have so many people to thank for getting me through the last seven years. I could never have done this alone. To all my aunts, uncles, and cousins who sent emails, cards, and gave us gifts in the beginning few years of James' life – we felt the love and support. To Kerstin for always being ready with a hug when we came home. To Keri for always caring, and for the phone call after James' first CT scan, and for crying on the phone with me that day. I obviously never forgot that ;) To some of the ladies at church back home who always took the time to check in with me, and who took the time to let me know they were praying for us – Norma, Hilda, Dolores, Sandy, Deb, Heather, Carol, Patty – you all touched my heart and encouraged me in a way that I won't forget.

To Kelly, who became a friend I will never lose touch with, for being someone who was always honest and real, even when things were raw and ugly. To Cheri, for being so much fun, and for your realness and willingness to step into my disaster, and for letting me into yours. We do disasters so well together! To Dolores, for becoming a friend in the midst of ugly things, and being someone that I strive to love like. To Ang, for your kind heart and easy laugh, and for the meal the day after James was diagnosed with cerebral palsy. You made chicken curry, and thankfully you hugged me when we got there and I got all my tears out then so I wasn't a blubbering mess all over your kitchen table.

To my brother and sister in law, for your genuine love of James which has always been so evident every time we get together. To my sister, who is usually the first to cry with me! And the first to show off her nephew in every situation! Thank you for your endless hugs and texts of encouragement, still to this day. Life wouldn't be nearly as fun without you to live it with.

To my inlaws, who have put together fundraisers in the beginning when we couldn't afford all that came with James and his needs. Thank you for seeing those practical needs. Thank you for your unconditional acceptance of us, and for all that you do to welcome us when we come home, and for all the efforts you make for your grandchildren.

To my parents, who have also accepted James for who he is, and are always looking for ways to help us. Thank you for your hospitality every time we are back for a whirlwind of appointments, and for your emotional support. Thank you for always greeting us with a hug, and sending us away with a hug.

To my best friend, Christine. Thank you for all the work you have put into us. Thank you for all of your time, for picking me up far more than anyone needs to know ;) For being a safe place for me to remember that I am a person outside of being a mom and a 24/7 care giver. For reminding me of all the things I loved before everything changed, and for encouraging me to pursue those things again. For inspiring me to do better every day, without pushing. Because we both know I don't like to be pushed. Thank you for the love you have shown me, and taught me. Thank you for letting me into your life, and trusting me on the same level that I have come to trust you. Thank you for being my person.

To my husband, thank you for staying. Thank you for staying when life felt like hell on earth, with no way out. Thank you for loving me when I was pretty unlovable. Thank you for being a phenomenal father to Julia and to James; and believe me, that requires two completely different skill sets, both of which you have. Thank you for your physical strength when I have struggled with James. Thank you for your emotional strength when I have been done and needed to step out. Thank you for your wisdom. Thank you for how hard you have worked so that I can stay home and do everything that James requires.

And how can I talk about relationships without talking about James' sister. The immense sacrifices that she has made along this road. Often times, people feel sorry for a child who is raised in a family with a dependent sibling. They see all that child has had to give up. And it is so true, they give up so much that most people will never see or understand. They also gain so much more that most children never have the privilege of learning.

Julia is two years older than James, and she has been over shadowed by him since the day he was born. In the first few years she was hauled hours away for appointments every week with him. She had to entertain herself while James screamed, needed to be fed constantly, had his hygiene taken care of, did daily physiotherapy, and the list goes on and on. Her bedtimes were rushed because James was screaming. Her mornings were lonely because I was falling asleep every second that I wasn't busy with James.

She didn't have a mommy who was able to spend hours at the kitchen table coloring and doing crafts. We did make it to the park, but not for very long because James was screaming. We didn't go on holidays for many years because there was just no point in going away to spend lots of money and still deal with the day and night crying. We didn't have a lot of money to buy her fancy toys, because

James' needs and appointments were so expensive, and we were a full time student family with no income beyond student loans.

She took on too much responsibility from the very beginning. She would run me blankets when James was puking in my arms. Every day. Now that she is nine, she runs to him with a blanket if I am not in the room and she takes care of him until I get there. She calls for me as soon as there are signs that he is going to start choking. She knows that we cannot be out late, as it interferes with his medications and sleeping.

She knows the signs when he is getting sick. He flutters his eyes weirdly and shutters. She knows that means he is likely going to be sick the next day. She knows that there is a difference between sick puke and choking puke.

She stands up for her brother and protects him. If a friend dares to judge James or say anything less than kind she is the first to speak up and defend him. And she not only defends him, she explains why he is doing what he is doing. She wants her friends to love him. They play hide and go seek with him now! One hides, and then James rats out where they are hiding by pointing and laughing once the other person comes looking.

Julia knows that when we go to the lake, we need both parents, or else she has to swim alone. If I take the kids alone, I bring a small inflatable boat for James. The lake water is too cold for him and he doesn't like it; so I lie him in there and tow him around behind me! This way I can be in the water with Julia, but I still can't really play the way she likes to play as I always have to be holding onto that boat.

Julia sees people with disabilities as valuable people, who maybe simply need some help to do things that other people take for granted. She is loud and demanding, but has also become a very observant and soft hearted young lady. She is able to see past everything that may be going on, to see that someone might be feeling sad. Or to see that maybe someone cannot participate because of a limitation. She doesn't act on that too much right now; she still likes to stick pretty close to me. But that compassion is there, and I am so excited to see how that develops.

Siblings of a dependent child live in a world that most do not understand. They sacrifice normal things every day. And while I try my hardest to consciously not give Julia more responsibility with James than she should have as a young girl, it just happens naturally. It is our family dynamic. They have a bond that is unspoken and so beautiful.

She likes to push him in his wheelchair when we go out. If he cries in the van she quietly reaches over and takes his hand and simply holds it so he doesn't feel alone. Or she makes up a game to play with him, so he laughs for the remainder of our trip. She makes blanket beds on the floor to cuddle with him and watch movies. We set up a railing on her bed and he has sleepovers in her room. She goes to visit him in school in his classroom just to say hi and see how he is doing. She looks for him on the playground to see if he is having fun.

For all that she has sacrificed I am so proud. And for all that her heart has gained I am so thankful. You cannot love James and not learn compassion.

Closing

It is time for me to wrap this all up. I hope that as you have walked through this journey with me, you have felt encouraged, no matter what path you are on.

If you are also raising a very dependent child, I hope that you feel less alone. That a piece of your heart found a piece of my heart through our story. My hope is that in moments you could identify with my heart. That all of your unspoken grief, anger, sadness, joys, triumphs, and failures feel like they have just a little bit more validation. That you feel like the day to day routine is bearable, because you are not alone.

If you are a caregiver in any capacity, I hope that you also feel less alone. Even though this may only be a calling for a time in your life, your heart fits right in with those of us who will be doing this for our lifetime. What a great responsibility you have taken on in the name of love. Know that to someone, you are everything. You are their only passage to the outside world. Their only source of dignity. You speak to them what their self worth is simply by how you choose to treat them and handle them. You can fill their heart, or you can break it, all in the way you care for their bodies.

If you have simply read this to get a glimpse into the life of a mom raising a dependent child, I thank you.

Thank you for taking these moments to hear my heart, and the heart of so many doing the very same things day in and day out. Thank you for the ways you may have allowed your heart to change. If this has ignited any sense of compassion for someone in your life who may be dependent upon others to get them through, please hold onto that until you know how to best put that to use. It could be something as simple as making eye contact with them the next time you are in the same room and saying good morning.

Raising James is the hardest thing I have ever been entrusted with. It stretches me and breaks me every day. It is exhausting beyond measure – physically, mentally, emotionally, spiritually. But James has taught me love, compassion, and true joy.

My goal was to let you into my heart, and encourage your heart in the midst of real everyday life. I hope that most of this has been encouraging and enlightening. But I also wanted to be real; real about the reality that while I have very willingly given the whole of my life to doing the very best that I can for James, my days can get dark. Very dark. It is something that is very common among other families doing much the same things every day, it just isn't talked about.

I so desperately want people to see the good in James. To see his love and joy. To want to be near him, to love being near him. I want the world to know the James that I know. But my daily reality is that I live in fear that I do not know my own son. I will never know him the way that he needs and deserves to be known. The grind of caring for his every need is grueling and isolating. My world gets dangerously dark when his health nose dives, when we cannot communicate successfully with him, when his body is rejecting basic nutrition time and time again. When I see him slowly falling off the cerebral palsy pediatric growth charts. When he screams for days and I can't do anything to help him. When the reality of what he was robbed of surfaces, almost daily.

    I just carried James to bed. And for the first time in a week, he stayed sleeping. He is now 118cm long, 47.5 pounds, with no centre of gravity. He is just two weeks shy of his eighth birthday as I write these final words. He is starting to make new vocal sounds, that sound much like "yaya" and "dada", and even uses that at appropriate times occasionally! His nutrition has changed yet again; he is now getting all nutrition by purees orally, and only milk and water through his tube. It feels as though he is changing so fast right now, and I am simply trying to keep up and keep doing what is best for him.
    My heart feels a burden that I rarely share. Thank you for sharing it with me.

I would love to hear from you once you have finished this book. Feel free to send me an email at jeepincj7ca@hotmail.com.